Food for Thought

VERNON C

CW00736288

Acataloguerecordforthisbookisavailablefromthe BritishLibrary.

The author

Vernon Coleman MB ChB DSc is a qualified medical practitioner with many years of experience as a GP. He is the author of over 100 other books, many of which are available as kindle books on Amazon. For a list of books please see Vernon Coleman's author page on Amazon or visit http://www.vernoncoleman.com/

CONTENTS

Food the fuel 1
Safe drinking..37
How healthy are your eating habits? 53
Food additives..57
How much do you know about food safety? 66
Drugs and hormones...78
Mad cow disease..84
Food irradiation – facts you should know 89
Microwave ovens..93
Genetically altered food..102
Foods that cause cancer 109
Foods to avoid — and foods to eat — to cut your cancer risk 140
Other common diseases — and their relationship to what you eat 157
Twenty one reasons for being a vegetarian 185
Healthy eating — step one: eat more fibre 202
Healthy eating — step two: eat less sugar 207
Healthy eating — step three: eat less fat 211
101 Superfoods 229
Overweight 248
How much should you weigh? 252
The dirty dozen: dieting myths 258
Ten dieting excuses — and why you should forget them..............266
Dr Vernon Coleman's slim for life programme 272
Forty eight quick tips for losing weight............................282
Children who are overweight 290

Warning

CHAPTER ONE

FOOD THE FUEL

In an average lifetime you will eat thirty tons of food.

From those thirty tons of food your body will derive the building materials it needs both to grow and to repair itself and the energy to keep muscles functioning and organs such as the brain and the liver operating effectively. Food helps to provide the fuel to keep you warm and to keep your heart pumping.

If you eat too much food then the excess will be turned into fat and stored. The idea of storing food as fat is that if at any time in the future your intake of food is less than your body needs then the stored fat can be used as a reserve supply.

The food that you eat is made up of carbohydrates, fats, proteins, vitamins and minerals.

Carbohydrates

Carbohydrates have a terrible reputation — particularly among slimmers who always regard them as a threat to dieting success. It is true that some carbohydrates are bad for you. But other carbohydrates are excellent and essential foodstuffs. If you are going to eat healthily you must know the difference between the good and the bad.

There are three basic types of carbohydrate:
* simple carbohydrates (also known as sugars)
* complex carbohydrates (also known as starches)
* fibre (also known as roughage)

Simple carbohydrates

These are the 'bad' carbohydrates — the ones your body can do without. They are full of calories and will provide you with a lot of energy — often very quickly — but by and large they don't contain

1

anything else of much value. Honey (which is basically a type of sugar) is very much a mysterious exception and some types of sugar (such as blackstrap molasses) contain a few minerals but basically sugar is something you can do without.

You should keep your intake of sugar down because sugar causes tooth decay, makes you fat and increases your risk of developing heart disease. There is even evidence now which shows that too much sugar may increase your chances of developing cancer.

Complex carbohydrates

Simple carbohydrates — sugars — are broken down very quickly in the body. That is why they provide more or less 'instant' energy. Complex carbohydrates — foods such as cereals, pasta, rice, pulses and fruits and vegetables — are digested much more slowly.

You should increase your intake of complex carbohydrates because foods that are rich in starch also tend to contain essentials such as protein, iron and vitamins. They are also often rich in fibre and usually contain relatively few calories. You can easily increase your intake of complex carbohydrates by eating more bread (just buy bread — preferably wholemeal — which tastes good and cut it thicker), more pasta (preferably wholemeal), more pulses (beans and peas), more rice (brown rice is better for you) and more fresh fruit and vegetables. Wholemeal bread and pasta and brown rice are better because they contain more fibre and haven't had so many of the original vitamins and minerals removed in the manufacturing process. Starchy foods contain a lot of potential energy and also contain a lot of the essential proteins, vitamins and minerals to enable your body to remain healthy and strong.

Fibre

Your body needs a plentiful and regular supply of roughage. The list of disorders known to be associated with a low fibre diet is constantly growing but already includes cancer, diverticular disease, gallstones, varicose veins and appendicitis. Fibre consists of a number of complex carbohydrates and there are two types: soluble fibre and insoluble fibre. Most foods which contain fibre include both types.

Soluble fibre has two important jobs. First, it forms a sticky substance in your stomach which restricts the amount of fat that your body absorbs from the other food you have eaten. Second, it helps to control the production of insulin (the hormone which controls the level of your blood sugar) and thereby helps to stop you feeling hungry. Soluble fibre is found in most vegetables and fruits, in oats, barley and rye and in pulses such as peas and beans.

Insoluble fibre is found in wheat (and in the bread and cereals which are made from them) and in some vegetables. As you might imagine from the fact that it is insoluble this type of fibre doesn't turn into a sticky mass but acts like a sponge and simply swells up as it absorbs the liquid in your stomach. It is because it swells up that insoluble fibre helps to make you feel full — and stops you eating so much.

Protein

Your body makes its own protein from the amino acids which are in the proteins you eat; it needs protein to grow and to repair damaged tissues. There are twenty two types of amino acid — all containing nitrogen — in your body. Eight of the amino acids which are used to create adult proteins and ten of the amino acids used to create proteins in children have to be obtained in our diet because our bodies cannot make them. These amino acids are, not surprisingly, known as 'essential' amino acids. Any good, balanced diet will contain all the amino acids your body needs — including these 'essential' amino acids.

You don't need to eat meat to get the amino acids your body needs to make protein. For example, soya beans, seeds and nuts all contain essential ingredients for making protein. Whatever type of protein rich food you eat the protein will be broken down into amino acids which will then be absorbed into your body. If your diet doesn't contain enough material to make proteins then the proteins already in your body — usually starting with the ones in your muscles — will be cannibalised to keep you alive. Your body cannot store protein in the same way that it can store fat and so you need a regular supply of protein. If you eat too much protein then the excess is excreted (although some of it will be converted into fat and stored as fat).

You must eat enough protein because:

1. If you eat too little protein then tissue proteins — particularly muscles — will be broken down.

2. Protein is essential for growth and for the repair of damaged tissues.

3. Protein is essential for the production of some enzymes.

But don't eat too much protein because:

1. If you eat more protein than your body needs the amino acids in the protein will be broken down and some of the protein will be converted into body fat.

2. Eating too much protein may also increase the loss of calcium from your body — with an increased risk of osteoporosis developing.

3. In addition too much protein may put a strain on your liver and kidneys.

4. Eating too much protein may lead to vitamin deficiency.

5. Too much protein may produce an increased risk of cancer and heart disease.

Fat

Fat has a terrible reputation. The bad image is well deserved. Fat in your diet can cause heart disease and high blood pressure and can increase your chances of having a stroke.

But some fat is essential and the bad reputation that fat has acquired is largely due to the fact that most people eat far too much of it. Many people get one half of their calorie intake from fat and most people would be healthier if they ate less fat and, in particular, if their consumption of saturated fat was reduced.

In practical terms this means cutting down on the consumption of meat and dairy produce such as milk, cream, butter and cheese for it is these foods which contain large amounts of saturated fat.

There are three types of fatty acid in fat: saturated, unsaturated and polyunsaturated. But different fats contain these three types in different proportions. Saturated fats cause trouble because our bodies cannot digest them properly. The result is that they stay in the blood for a long time, sticking to the inside of the blood vessels. In the end these sticky, indigestible saturated fats clog up the blood vessels — producing a condition called atherosclerosis which leads to high blood pressure, heart disease and stroke. Saturated fats also interfere with the metabolism of other foods and with the removal of wastes. Polyunsaturated fats are much healthier and much more useful.

You can often tell which sort of fat a food contains by looking at it. Foods like butter and lard which are rich in saturated fatty acids are hard at room temperature. Foods containing unsaturated fatty acids tend to be liquid or oily. It is healthier to cook with liquid fats such as sunflower oil or safflower oil (which are rich in polyunsaturated fatty acids) than to cook with solid fats such as lard or butter. (But watch out: palm oil and coconut oil are both plant oils but they do contain quite a lot of saturated fat.)

Cholesterol

Cholesterol, which is present in all animal tissues, has some similar properties to fat but is recognised as being potentially dangerous because if the level of cholesterol in your blood reaches too high a concentration then it may increase your chances of having a heart attack.

Cholesterol is present in many ordinary foods (cheese, chocolate, cream, eggs, heart, kidneys, liver, crab, lobster, brains, caviar) but most of the cholesterol in our bodies comes not from foods that contain cholesterol itself but from other fatty foods.

Your body can make its own cholesterol from saturated fats so if your diet contains a high quantity of saturated fat then your body will make more cholesterol and your blood cholesterol level will probably rise. (Unsaturated fats provide the same amount of energy as saturated fats but tend to reduce blood cholesterol levels.)

Vitamins and minerals

Although they are sometimes called 'micro-nutrients' because we need them in such very small quantities, vitamins and minerals are essential for healthy living.

Vitamins help keep your body tissues healthy, maintain your skin in good condition, produce enzymes to enable your body to function, help turn food into energy, keep your nerves in good condition, assist in the production of hormones, help keep your teeth and bones strong and aid in the production of blood cells.

Minerals also play a vital part in the functioning of your body. For example, iron is essential for the formation of red blood cells. If your body is deficient in iron then your body will form too few red blood cells — the cells which normally carry oxygen around your body — and your tissues will not receive enough oxygen. Calcium helps form the structure of your bones and teeth. Zinc is essential for the proper functioning of some of your body's enzymes.

For the last two decades there has been a considerable amount of discussion about the value of vitamins (particularly vitamins A and C) in the prevention — and even treatment — of cancer. In vitamin A it is the beta-carotene content which is believed to have the protective quality. Researchers have found that people who eat a diet which is low in vitamin A tend to be more likely to suffer from cancers of the lung, larynx, bladder, oesophagus, stomach, colon, rectum and prostate. And it has been found that vitamin C may lower the risk of cancer of the oesophagus and stomach.

Vitamins aren't the only micronutrients which help prevent cancer. Minerals can play a part too. Zinc, for example, is believed to help prevent cancer. I am aware of three scientific papers which have shown that there may be a link between a low zinc intake and prostate cancer.

7

Despite all the billions of dollars spent on research no one yet knows how cancer develops. One theory is that free radicals — molecules produced routinely within the body — may damage the DNA within our cells, transforming a previously normal cell into a potentially cancerous cell. Every cell in the human body needs oxygen but oxygen is responsible for the production of free radicals — oxygen carrying molecules which are destructive and aggressive. It is free radicals which encourage our tissues and bodies to age and which cause damage to cells and tissues when our immune systems falter. The formation of free radicals is an inevitable part of life. (And is added to by pollutants from the outside world. For example, a smoker breathes in several billion free radicals every time he sucks on a cigarette.)

Fortunately, it is now believed that there are some food substances called anti-oxidants which can neutralise free radicals which are formed. There are four known anti-oxidants at the moment: beta-carotene (which is converted in the human body to vitamin A), vitamins C and E and the mineral selenium. There is a growing amount of evidence to show that anti-oxidants can help reduce the likelihood of numerous diseases including: cancer, arteriosclerosis, heart disease, skin diseases, types of arthritis, Parkinson's disease, cataracts, Alzheimer's disease and radiation damage. The anti-oxidants could, it seems, even help to counter the effects of ageing.

Finally, it is worth pointing out that human experiments have shown that your body can repair the DNA which has been damaged by free radicals if it receives a plentiful supply of folic acid — one of the vitamin B complex of vitamins. Your body will receive the folic acid it needs if you eat a diet which is rich in dark green, leafy vegetables, fruits, dried peas, beans and wheatgerm.

BE CAREFUL HOW YOU PREPARE YOUR FOOD

It is important to be careful about how you store and prepare your food. Vitamin C and the vitamins in the B group are water soluble, which makes them especially vulnerable. As well as being very sensitive to heat, they leach out of food when it is soaked, blanched or boiled. Put a cabbage into cold water and bring it to the boil and you destroy 75% of its vitamin C content. Cook fresh peas for just five minutes and you wipe out 20-40% of their thiamine (one of the B vitamins) and 30-40% of their vitamin C.

Other B vitamins especially at risk in vegetables are folate, and riboflavin. Folic acid is sensitive to heat and light and it is soluble in water. If you boil your vegetables in too much water, cook food at too high a temperature or even allow your lettuce to soak in water for too long then much of the folic acid will be lost.

Even before you start cooking you can damage the vitamin content of food simply by keeping it for too long. If salad, spinach or green beans or peas are stored for a day they lose up to 40% of their vitamin C content. After another day in storage they may lose the same amount again. If salad vegetables are allowed to stand in water for a quarter of an hour they may lose up to 30% of their vitamin C content and a considerable amount of the vitamin B1 content.

Vitamins are also lost when food is cut up. And the more you chop food the greater the vitamin loss. If bananas or tomatoes are allowed to stand after being chopped they lose 10% of their vitamin content within minutes. Chopped red cabbage may lose 60% of its vitamin content if allowed to stand for two hours. (Incidentally, dribbling a little vinegar or lemon juice onto freshly prepared food may help to slow down the loss of vitamin C.) When fruit is peeled and potatoes and tomatoes skinned most of the vitamins are lost.

Vitamins A, D, E and K are fat soluble and so less at risk. Nevertheless, up to 50% of the vitamin E in food can be destroyed by frying or baking and the A vitamin and carotene are destroyed at high temperatures.

Making sure that you get the best out of the food you eat is not difficult: it simply requires a little knowledge and a little care. Modern raw foodstuffs are not intrinsically worthless; they are more likely to be emptied of essential vitamins and minerals by careless preparation in the home and the kitchen than by having been grown in poor soil.

Vitamin and Mineral Fact File

VITAMIN A (RETINOL)

What It Does:

Although vitamin A is probably best known as the vitamin that helps us to see in the dark, this reputation is rather exaggerated. The fact is that an excess of vitamin A won't help you see better — vitamin A does help us to see in dim light and a deficiency can cause night blindness but that's about as far as it goes. Another important function of vitamin A is to help us fight infection. Anyone deficient in vitamin A will be more susceptible to infection. Since vitamin A is an anti-oxidant a shortage of vitamin A may lead to the development of certain types of cancer. Vitamin A may also help protect against heart disease and is necessary for sexual function. Vitamin A also helps in the formation of bones and teeth and helps to keep skin and hair healthy.

Where You May Find It:

Some animal foods — for example, liver, eggs and butter — are particularly rich in vitamin A and are sometimes said to be a suitable source of the vitamin. There are, however, two big problems with animal sources of vitamin A. First, the animal foods which are rich in vitamin A are also often rich in fat. Dairy products rich in fat, such as milk, cheese, butter and ice cream, are rich in vitamin A but are also likely to block your arteries and lead to the development of heart disease and cancer. Second, some animal products are so rich in vitamin A that they can be dangerous.

Retinol is only found in animal foods but the carotenes, of which the most important is beta-carotene, are found in carrots and other orange and yellow/orange fruits and vegetables and dark green, leafy vegetables. In the body, beta-carotene is converted to vitamin A. Unlike retinol, foods which contain beta-carotene can be consumed in plentiful amounts without fear of toxicity. You can obtain all the Vitamin A you need from plant foods.

Good supplies of beta-carotene can be obtained from carrots, broccoli, chicory, endives, spinach, lettuce, apricots, elderberries and mangoes. Other useful sources include: sweet potatoes, pumpkin, peas, spinach, kale, peppers, melons, cabbage, peaches, asparagus, watermelon, tomatoes, parsley, avocado. The average person has a two year supply of vitamin A stored in their liver.

Possible Signs of Deficiency May Include:
Night blindness; lack of tear secretion; changes in eyes with eventual blindness if deficiency is severe and untreated; increased susceptibility to respiratory infection; dry, rough skin; changes in mucous membranes; weight loss; poor bone growth; weak tooth enamel; diarrhoea; slow growth.

Possible Signs Of Overdose/Toxicity May Include:

A high intake of retinol — the animal form of vitamin A — can be harmful, causing liver and bone damage. Anorexia, drowsiness, irritability, hair loss, headaches and skin problems are possible symptoms. Excessive consumption by pregnant women of vitamin A, but not beta-carotene, has also been linked with an increased risk of birth defects. Children are more sensitive to vitamin A and are more likely to develop toxicity with high dosages. Taking oral contraceptives may increase vitamin A concentration.

VITAMIN B

Note: When vitamins were first discovered they were given letters as they were discovered — A, B, C, D etc. But scientists then discovered that the substance they had called vitamin B actually consisted of several different substances, so they began to rename the vitamins in the B group, calling them B1, B2, B3 and so on. To add to the confusion some of the vitamins in the B group — are also known by names. Vitamin B1, for example, is known as thiamine while vitamin B2 is sometimes called riboflavin.

VITAMIN B1 (THIAMINE)

What It Does:

Vitamin B1 is used by the body to release energy from carbohydrates, fats and alcohol. The bigger the carbohydrate consumption the greater the need for thiamine. This can lead to deficiency if high levels of refined carbohydrate are eaten.

Where You May Find It:

Vitamin B1 is present in many different plant foods but most of us get all the vitamin B1 we need from the cereals we eat. As with rice much of the vitamin B1 is removed from the husk during the milling process. Theoretically, therefore, white flour should be deficient in vitamin B1. However, most countries have laws which ensure that white flour has the missing vitamin B1 put back into it. Foods which contain vitamin B1 include: peas, wholewheat flour, wheatgerm, dried sunflower seeds, brown rice, soya beans, kidney beans.

Possible Signs of Deficiency May Include:

If your body is short of vitamin B1 then you are likely to develop fairly typical symptoms which consist of numbness and pins and needles in your hands and feet. A severe deficiency of vitamin B1 can lead to a condition called beri-beri which is particularly common in rice-eating countries where the husk (the part of the rice which contains vitamin B1) is removed and the rice is polished.

Deficiency of thiamine may also cause palpitations and muscular weakness; loss of appetite; anorexia; indigestion; constipation; fatigue; nausea and vomiting; depression and other mental problems such as memory loss and personality changes. Vitamin B1 deficiency is common among alcoholics and elderly people — particularly those who live alone and may not feed themselves properly. In alcoholics vitamin B1 deficiency can lead to permanent brain damage. In the elderly vitamin B1 deficiency commonly leads to mental confusion and to heart disease.

Possible Signs of Overdose/Toxicity May Include:

The vitamins in the vitamin B group can cause a wide range of problems when taken in excess (despite the fact that vitamin B, like vitamin C, is water soluble and therefore excesses of the vitamin are eventually discarded in the urine).

Occasionally large doses of vitamin B1 have caused hypersensitive reactions resembling anaphylactic shock. The vitamin may cause drowsiness in some people.

VITAMIN B2 (RIBOFLAVIN)

What It Does:

Vitamin B2 helps your body turn carbohydrate foodstuffs into energy. (It shares this duty with vitamin B1 and vitamin B3). It isn't particularly easy to become deficient in vitamin B2 but if you do then your first symptoms are likely to include sore, cracked lips and a sore, discoloured tongue. When vitamin B2 deficiency does occur it is usually accompanied by a deficiency of other vitamins. Vitamin B2 also helps keeps the eyes healthy, and helps keep the skin, tongue and mouth healthy. It helps preserve the nervous system and promotes normal growth and development.

Where You May Find It:

Vitamin B2 is found in fairly large quantities in eggs and in dairy products such as milk and cheese; however, since vitamin B2 is sensitive to light the vitamin B2 content of milk can be destroyed if the milk is left in full sunshine on the doorstep. Vitamin B2 is also found in wholemeal products and wheatgerm, broccoli, spinach and brewer's yeast.

Possible Signs Of Deficiency May Include:

Cracks and sores in the corners of mouth and inflammation of tongue and lips. The eyes become red, sore, sensitive to light and easily tired, there is itching and scaling of skin around the nose, mouth, forehead, ears and scalp. Other symptoms may include: trembling; dizziness; tiredness; poor concentration; insomnia.

Possible Signs Of Overdose/Toxicity May Include:

Dark urine; nausea; vomiting.

VITAMIN B3 (NIACIN — CONSISTING OF NICOTINIC ACID AND NICOTINAMIDE)

What It Does:

Vitamin B3 helps turn food into energy and helps to maintain the skin, nerves and digestive system.

Where You May Find It:
Vitamin B3 can be found m a wide variety of plant and animal foods. Liver, chicken and fish contain it. Sunflower seeds, nuts and many vegetable and cereal foodstuffs contain it.

Possible Signs Of Deficiency May Include:
Muscle weakness; general fatigue; loss of appetite; headaches; swollen, red tongue; skin lesions, including rashes; dry scaly skin; wrinkles; coarse skin texture; nausea and vomiting; dermatitis; diarrhoea, irritability; dizziness. A severe deficiency can cause a disorder called pellagra — this will affect the brain, skin and gastro-intestinal tract and can result in death.

Possible Signs Of Overdose/Toxicity May Include:
Nausea; vomiting; abdominal cramps; diarrhoea; weakness; light-headedness; headache; fainting; sweating; high blood sugar; heart-rhythm disturbances; jaundice.

VITAMIN B5 (PANTOTHENIC ACID)

What It Does:
Promotes normal growth and development; aids in release of energy from fats, carbohydrates and proteins and helps the synthesis of numerous body materials.

Where You May Find It:
A diet with a good nutritional intake of the other B group vitamins will contain enough vitamin B5. (Sources include offal, meat and cereals.)

Possible Signs Of Deficiency May Include:

Vitamin B5 is so widely distributed in foods that deficiency is rare.

Possible Signs Of Overdose/Toxicity May Include:
Diarrhoea and water retention.

VITAMIN B6 (PYRIDOXINE)

What It Does:
Vitamin B6 plays a vital role in the way enzymes metabolize proteins and amino acids. However, although some drugs (notably the oral contraceptives) increase the human body's requirement for vitamin B6, diseases due to vitamin B6 deficiency are not usually reported in adult human beings. The body's requirement for vitamin B6 increases with protein consumption — and, in particular, with the consumption of animal protein. Meat-eaters have a greater need for this vitamin than vegetarians and vegans.

Where You May Find It:
No particular foods contain large amounts of vitamin B6 but many foods contain small amounts and your body's requirements for the vitamin are small. Meat, offal, fruit, vegetables and cereals contain vitamin B6. Foods containing vitamin B6 include: bananas, potatoes, peas, carrots, cabbage and beans, cereal products and bread.

Possible Signs Of Deficiency May Include:
Weakness; mental confusion or depression; irritability; hyperactivity; skin lesions and anaemia.

Possible Signs of Overdose/Toxicity May Include:
Too much vitamin B6 can cause depression and nerve damage that can lead to clumsiness, numbness and a loss of balance.

VITAMIN B9 (FOLIC ACID)

Note: the word 'folate' is a generic term for the many compounds which are derived from folic acid.

What It Does:

Promotes normal red blood cell formation and is essential for protein metabolism. Recent research suggests that people who have a diet which is low in folic acid may be more likely to die of heart disease.

Where You May Find It:

In green, leafy vegetables, such as spinach, kale, lettuce and also in wholemeal products, peas, rice and soya beans.

Possible Signs Of Deficiency May Include:

Anaemia; infertility; abnormalities of the linings of the intestines, vagina, uterus and bronchi.

Possible Signs Of Overdose/Toxicity May Include:

Appetite loss; nausea; flatulence.

VITAMIN B12 (CYANOCOBALAMIN)

What It Does:

Like folic acid, vitamin B12 is essential for the formation of red blood cells. If your body is short of vitamin B12 you are likely to develop a condition called pernicious anaemia — the size of your individual red blood cells will be increased but their number will be reduced. Vitamin B12 plays a vital part in the working of your central nervous system. A long term shortage of the vitamin can lead to permanent damage being done to the brain and spinal cord. Vitamin B12 aids the production of genetic matter inside cells which is needed for the creation of new cells. Vitamin B12 is an unusual vitamin in that before it can be absorbed into the body it needs to be linked to a substance called 'intrinsic factor' which is formed in the stomach. Patients who have had stomach surgery may be unable to produce this 'intrinsic factor'. This problem is less common these days now that ulcer healing drugs have made many stomach operations obsolete.

Where You May Find It:

Found in many animal products — including meat, eggs and dairy produce. Also available in tempeh, soya milk, edible seaweeds, dried spirulina and the wide range of fortified products now available (including cereals, margarines, textured vegetable proteins and fortified yeast extracts and savoury spreads). Vitamin B12 is manufactured by micro-organisms such as yeasts, bacteria, moulds and some algae.

The human body can store this vitamin for long periods (up to five or six years) so a daily dietary source is therefore not necessary. In addition, the healthy body recycles this vitamin very effectively, recovering it from bile and other intestinal secretions, which is why the dietary requirement is so low. There is also some evidence that vitamin B12 may be produced by bacterial activity in the small intestine.

Vitamin B12 is also found in nutritional yeast, beer, cider, fermented soya foods (such as soy sauce), barley malt syrup and parsley. The most reliable vegan sources of B12 are foods fortified with the vitamin. Soya products (such as soya milks), breakfast cereals, yeast extracts and margarines are particularly likely to contain added vitamin B12.

Vegan women who are pregnant and vegan mothers who intend to breast feed their babies should make sure that they eat foods which are fortified with vitamin B12 and they should talk to their doctors too.

Possible Signs Of Deficiency May Include:

Pernicious anaemia with the following symptoms: fatigue; weakness, especially in arms and legs; sore tongue; nausea; appetite loss; weight loss; bleeding gums; numbness and tingling in hands and feet; difficulty in maintaining balance; pale lips; pale tongue; pale gums; yellow eyes and skin; shortness of breath; depression; confusion and dementia; headache; poor memory. First obvious signs of B12 deficiency might be pins and needles or coldness in the hands and feet, fatigue and weakness, poor concentration or even psychosis.

Possible Signs Of Overdose/Toxicity May Include:
If taken with large doses of vitamin C, vitamin B12 may cause nose bleeding, ear bleeding, dry mouth.

VITAMIN H (B-GROUP VITAMIN, BIOTIN)

What It Does:
Essential for normal growth and development and repair and for a healthy metabolism.

Where You May Find It:
Intestinal bacteria probably produce all the biotin the body needs. The vitamin is available in almost all foods including brown rice, bulgur wheat, cashew nuts, peas, lentils, oats, soya beans, sunflower seeds.

Possible Signs Of Deficiency May Include:
Dry scaly dermatitis; nausea and vomiting; anorexia; fatigue; depression; sleepiness; muscular pains; loss of muscular reflexes; tongue becomes smooth and pale; hair loss; anaemia.

Possible Signs Of Overdose/Toxicity May Include:
Unlikely.

VITAMIN C (ASCORBIC ACID)

What It Does:

Vitamin C helps the body to form connective tissue — the packing material which supports and protects the rest of the body. Your skin contains a considerable amount of connective tissue and if you are short of vitamin C the first symptoms you notice are likely to be bruising and bleeding. This condition is called scurvy and the gums are usually the first part of the body to show it. In addition small cuts and grazes take an extraordinarily long time to heal. Scurvy is still fairly common — usually among people who do not eat enough fresh fruit and vegetables.

Vitamin C also helps your body to fight off infections and it helps your body to absorb iron. Indeed vitamin C increases the ease with which iron is absorbed by a factor of five. Meat eaters are often more likely to develop iron deficiency anaemia because they tend to eat less fruit and vegetables.

Vitamin C also helps the body to use calcium to build bones and blood vessels. Women need slightly more vitamin C than men and the sick and convalescent need good supplies of vitamin C in order to get well again. We need regular supplies of vitamin C since, like all the vitamins in the B group, it is water soluble.

Where You May Find It:

Fresh fruit of most kinds (but particularly citrus fruits) and fresh vegetables contain good quantities of vitamin C. One of the most important sources of vitamin C, however, is the potato (simply because it is such an important constituent in our diets). New potatoes contain more vitamin C than old ones and overcooking potatoes destroys the vitamin.

Since vitamin C is water soluble, leaving vegetables to soak in water for a long time will cause the vitamin C to disappear. Vitamin C is extremely fragile. It is destroyed by heat and it leaks out of foods into the water in which they are being cooked.

Possible Signs Of Deficiency May Include:
Wounds fail to heal and there is an increased liability to infection. Severe deficiency manifests as scurvy: muscle weakness; swollen gums; loss of teeth; tiredness; depression; bleeding under skin; bleeding gums.

Possible Signs Of Overdose/Toxicity May Include:
Large amounts of vitamin C can produce diarrhoea and gastric irritation and it is possible that too much vitamin C may cause kidney problems — specifically kidney stones — and can affect growing bones. In addition people who have been taking high doses of vitamin C for long periods and then suddenly cut down their intake can develop rebound scurvy.

VITAMIN D (CHOLECALCIFEROL, CALCIFEROL)

What It Does:
Vitamin D helps the body absorb and use calcium and phosphorus effectively for making strong bones and teeth. If your body is deficient in vitamin D then you will develop a condition called osteomalacia — in which your bones become weak and prone to fracture. In children a shortage of vitamin D leads to a condition called rickets.

Where You May Find It:
Your body can make its own vitamin D with the aid of a little sunshine and there are relatively few countries in the world where the supply of sunshine is inadequate for the manufacture of vitamin

D. Regular exposure of hands, arms and face to summer sunlight (for as little as ten to twenty minutes a day three times a week) can provide sufficient vitamin D. People with dark skin, or those who live in cloudy or smoggy areas or in northern areas, may need slightly more exposure.

The main dietary sources are fortified foods such as margarine and breakfast cereals although vitamin D is present in quite a number of different foods — salt water fish, mushrooms and dairy products for example.

Possible Signs Of Deficiency May Include:
Rickets (a childhood disease): bent, bowed legs; malformations of joints and bones. Osteomalacia (adult rickets): pain in ribs, lower spine, pelvis and legs; brittle, easily broken bones.

Possible Signs Of Overdose/Toxicity May Include:
Vitamin D, even in only relatively high doses, can damage the body by encouraging deposits of calcium. Vitamin D is one of the most toxic of vitamins when taken in excessive quantities.

VITAMIN E (TOCOPHEROL)

What It Does:
Vitamin E deficiency disorders are virtually unknown. Some manufacturers (and some fans of the vitamin) claim that vitamin E supplements can be used to boost mental, athletic or even sexual skills but I have not been able to find any scientific evidence to support these claims. Vitamin E has, over the years, acquired something of a reputation as a 'sex vitamin' but this reputation was based on experiments done on rats many decades ago. The experiments showed that a vitamin E deficiency in rats can lead to sterility. However, since a deficiency of vitamin E in human beings

is virtually unknown (you would probably have symptoms of something else before doctors identified a vitamin E deficiency if you were eating an inadequate diet) and since experiments on animals are of absolutely no value to human beings this evidence is clearly of no significance. More recently it has been claimed that vitamin E may help reduce the incidence of heart disease and may improve the immune system. This is far more likely. Vitamin E is an important anti-oxidant and therefore protects cells from damage by scavenging free radicals.

Where You May Find It:
Vitamin E is found in vegetable oils such as olive oil, sunflower oil and soya bean oil and in vegetables such as spinach, celery and broccoli. A vegetarian diet is particularly rich in vitamin E.

Possible Signs Of Deficiency May Include:
Lethargy; inability to concentrate; irritability; poor reflexes; visual disturbances; muscle weakness.

Possible Signs Of Overdose/Toxicity May Include:
Tendency to bleed; altered immunity; impaired sex functions; increased risk of blood clots; altered metabolism of essential hormones.

VITAMIN K (NAPTHAQUINONE)

What It Does:
Vitamin K plays an essential role in the blood clotting mechanism. It is rare for a healthy adult to be short of this vitamin since vitamin K is widely available in foods.

Where You May Find It:
In many vegetables, particularly green vegetables such as broccoli, cabbage, lettuce and spinach. Vitamin K is also produced by

bacterial activity in the large intestine. The use of antibiotics, which reduce gut bacteria, can occasionally cause deficiency.

Possible Signs of Deficiency May Include:
Excessive bleeding and haemorrhaging.

Possible Signs Of Overdose/Toxicity May Include:
Large doses may impair liver function.

Minerals and trace elements

CALCIUM

What It Does:
Helps build and maintain bones and teeth (99% of the calcium in the body is in the bones and teeth); controls transmission of nerve impulses; aids in muscle contraction; assists with blood clotting.

Where You May Find It:
Dairy products (such as milk and cheese) are sometimes thought of as a standard or irreplaceable source of calcium. However, this isn't true. For example, only about 30% of the calcium in milk is absorbed by the human body — possibly less than for typical green, leafy vegetables. Dark green, leafy vegetables (such as kale and broccoli) are good plant sources, and some experts believe that calcium is more readily absorbed from kale than it is from milk.

One recent study has shown that vegetarians absorb and retain more calcium from foods than do non-vegetarians and other studies cite lower rates of osteoporosis in vegetarians than in non-vegetarians. Vegetarian and vegan diets may actually protect against osteoporosis. The wisest course is to obtain dietary calcium from a wide range of sources. Possible calcium sources include: broccoli, molasses, chick peas, dried figs, tofu, endive, cabbage, kale, turnip greens, spinach and many different types of beans (including soya beans and baked beans). Probably the simplest way to make sure you get plenty of calcium is to eat plenty of dark green, leafy vegetables.

It is important to remember that a high calcium intake alone will not necessarily prevent osteoporosis. Countries where there is a high calcium intake (such as Sweden or Finland) tend to have higher fracture rates than countries (such as those in Asia) where calcium intake is not high. Apart from ensuring a reasonable intake of calcium it is necessary to reduce the loss of calcium from your body. There are six things you can do to minimise calcium loss:

1. Avoid tobacco (smokers have a hip fracture risk 40% higher than non-smokers).

2. Don't drink more than two cups of coffee a day.

3. Keep your intake of alcohol down.

4. Cut animal proteins out of your diet — this can slice your calcium losses in half.

5. Take regular, gentle exercise which you enjoy. (But do not exercise if it is painful and always consult your doctor before starting an exercise programme or altering your exercise habits.)

6. Keep your salt intake down.

Possible Signs Of Deficiency May Include:
Muscle spasms, such as leg cramps; high blood pressure.

Possible Signs Of Toxicity/Overdose May Include:

Confusion; high blood pressure; irregular heartbeat; depression; bone pain; muscle pain; nausea; vomiting; sensitivity of skin and eyes to light.

COPPER

What It Does:
Helps with production of red blood cells and controls enzyme activity which stimulates the formation of connective tissues and pigments which protect the skin.

Where You May Find It:
Wheatgerm, oats, peas, lentils, nuts and seeds. Also in liver, shellfish, dried beans, mushrooms, grapes.

Possible Signs Of Deficiency May Include:
Anaemia and a low white blood cell count associated with reduced resistance to infection.

Possible Signs Of Overdose/Toxicity May Include:
Nausea; vomiting; muscle aches; anaemia; abdominal pain. In some countries the amount of copper in drinking water has been enough to produce toxic effects.

IODINE

What It Does
Iodine helps produce thyroid hormones which control the rate of metabolism and control growth and development.

Where You May Find It:
Sunflower seeds, table salt (iodised), cod, haddock, shellfish. Levels in foods depend upon amount of iodine in the soil.

Possible Signs Of Deficiency May Include:

Listlessness (low thyroid hormone level); enlargement of the thyroid gland. Severe deficiency leads to cretinism in new born.

Possible Signs Of Overdose/Toxicity May Include:

Irregular heartbeat; confusion; swollen neck or throat; bloody .or black, tarry stools.

IRON

What It Does:

Helps with transport of oxygen from lungs to tissue and transports and stores oxygen in muscles; acts with production of essential enzymes.

Where You May Find It:

Iron is found in meat, fish and eggs but also in many vegetarian foods including green, leafy vegetables, nuts, cereals and beans. Foods rich in vitamin C eaten at the same time as iron-containing food will considerably increase absorption. Some of those who advocate meat eating claim that vegetarians are likely to have a diet which is deficient in iron. This is nonsense. A good, well-balanced vegetarian diet will contain plenty of iron.

Possible Signs Of Deficiency May Include:

Pale appearance; listlessness; fatigue; irritability.

Possible Signs Of Overdose/Toxicity May Include:

Too much iron may be as dangerous as too little. A vegetarian diet which allows the body to absorb the right amount of iron from several natural sources is probably the healthiest option. Iron supplements need to be taken with care; they can kill adults and children.

MAGNESIUM

What It Does:

Helps bones develop and helps nerves and muscles to function.

Where You May Find It:

It is an essential constituent of chlorophyll — and therefore green produce. Also found in whole grains, yeast extracts and nuts.

Possible Signs Of Deficiency May Include:

Muscle contractions; irritability; confusion.

Possible Signs Of Overdose/Toxicity May Include:

Severe nausea and vomiting; low blood pressure; muscle weakness; difficulty in breathing; heartbeat irregularity.

POTASSIUM

What It Does:

Maintains normal heart rhythm; helps in the generation of nerve impulses; helps with muscle contraction; controls body's water balance.

Where You May Find It:

In green, leafy vegetables, whole grain cereals and bread. Also in avocado, bananas, citrus fruits, juices (grapefruit, tomato, orange), lentils, molasses, many nuts, parsnips, dried peaches, potatoes, raisins.

Possible Signs Of Deficiency May Include:

Weakness; paralysis; low blood pressure; irregular or rapid heartbeat that can lead to cardiac arrest and death.

Possible Signs Of Overdose/Toxicity May Include:

Irregular or fast heartbeat; paralysis of arms and legs; blood pressure drop; convulsions; coma; cardiac arrest.

SELENIUM

What It Does:

Works as an anti-oxidant to protect cells from free radicals. May help preserve the elasticity of tissues.

Where You May Find It:

The selenium content in foods is closely related to the selenium content of the soil in which it is grown, which makes generalisations about the selenium content of foods difficult. But deficiency is not common, especially in countries where foods come from a wide variety of sources.

Foods likely to contain selenium include: meat, fish, shellfish, whole grain cereals, broccoli, dairy products.

Possible Signs Of Deficiency May Include:

A mild deficiency may affect the body's ability to deal with free radicals — and increase a risk of disorders including cancer. Gross deficiency may result in damage to the heart.

Possible Signs Of Overdose/Toxicity May Include:

Liver and heart disease; hair loss; nail loss; decaying teeth; fatigue; nausea; vomiting.

SODIUM

What It Does:

Maintains normal heart rhythm; controls body's water balance; helps with muscle contraction; helps with the generation of nerve impulses.

Where You May Find It:

Processed foods, smoked meat and fish. Also added in cooking and as table salt. Most people take far more sodium than they need.

Possible Signs Of Deficiency May Include:

Nausea; fatigue; muscle cramps; apathy; muscle twitching; appetite loss.

Possible Signs Of Overdose/Toxicity May Include:

Fluid retention, tissue swelling, coma.

ZINC

What It Does:

Zinc is essential for the functioning of many enzymes; it is also needed for wound healing and is a factor in many other vital processes. Enables growth and sexual development to occur.

Where You May Find It:

Whole grain cereals, wholemeal bread, wheat germ, sunflower seeds, soya beans. Also found in lean meat, fish, oysters and eggs.

Possible Signs Of Deficiency May Include:

Diminution of taste and smell; prolonged wound healing; reduced growth in children; loss of hair; inflammation of tongue, mouth, eyelids; reduced sperm count. Severe depletion results in dwarfism, small testicles, and enlarged spleen/liver.

Possible Signs Of Overdose/Toxicity May Include:

Drowsiness; lethargy; light-headedness; staggering gait; restlessness; repeated vomiting may lead to dehydration.

HOW TO PREPARE FOOD TO PRESERVE THE VITAMIN AND MINERAL CONTENT

Vitamins can easily be destroyed. Mushrooms, lettuce, broccoli, asparagus and strawberries, for example, all lose their vitamins very quickly. Food which has to be cooked should be cooked for the shortest possible time and at the lowest possible temperature.

In order to ensure that the food you eat retains a high vitamin content follow these simple rules:

1. Food processing tends to reduce the nutritional quality of food and so where possible you should try to buy fresh food and either eat it raw (if appropriate) or eat it after cooking for the shortest length of time.

2. Buy vegetables whole. Don't have the leaves removed from carrots or the stalk removed from a cabbage or cauliflower. If you buy the vegetable whole vitamin C will continue to be produced and moved into the edible parts of the plant.

3. Cook foods in the minimum amount of water or steam.

4. Avoid high cooking temperatures and long heat exposure.

5. Do not allow food to stand for long periods at room temperature. Do not store food in warm places.

6. Do not soak vegetables for long periods.

7. Do not peel fruit or vegetables unless necessary. (For example, do not peel apples or skin potatoes.)

8. Try to use food the day you have bought it rather than use frozen foods. Use foods the day you buy them to get the best out of them.

9. You can keep fresh products for longer by freezing as soon as you buy them. Deep freezing preserves vitamins and other nutrients. Vegetables should be blanched before freezing. Put them in hot

water for a short time. This inactivates enzymes which might otherwise degrade vitamin C.

10. Do not allow food — particularly unpackaged fruit and vegetables, vegetable oils and milk — to stand in sunlight.

ARE VITAMIN AND MINERAL SUPPLEMENTS NECESSARY?

For over a quarter of a century I was the most vocal and consistent critic of vitamin and mineral supplements. But I always added a rider to my criticism. I always promised that I would keep the situation under constant review and if I ever felt that vitamin and mineral supplements were necessary then I would say so. Changing an opinion is, in my view, a sign of strength not weakness.

A fundamental foundation stone for my argument over the years has always been my belief that it is much better (both more effective and safer) to take your needed vitamins and minerals in the food you eat than in an artificial way.

I have great faith in the ability of the human body to obtain what it needs from natural sources — to protect itself from a wide range of threats and to heal itself when necessary. But the world has changed. And I am convinced that the body now does need some outside help.

I believe that it will very soon be difficult (if not impossible) to obtain good quality food which contains the necessary basic ingredients for healthy living. It is already difficult to buy decent food. Supermarkets are very patchy suppliers of organic foods.

The food industry has recently introduced a number of techniques which are clearly not going to go away. Those of us who care about what we eat have, quite simply, lost the battle. I am not being defeatist in saying this: merely practical. There comes a time when one has to step back, take a good hard look at the situation and recognise the need to establish a new position from which to fight. We have lost a good many battles in recent years. But we have not yet lost the war.

Moreover, there is, I believe, a very real chance that the quality of organic food will deteriorate dramatically in the next year or two. The American food Goliaths are keen to dilute the meaning of the phrase 'organic food' and, sooner or later, I believe that they will succeed.

Unless you grow your own food (or obtain it from a neighbour) the chances are that within a few years the only food available (whether or not it is labelled as 'organic') will contain a rich mixture of hormones, chemicals, drug residues and other possible carcinogens.

Our bodies are now constantly under siege from a hostile world. And things are going to get worse.

Microwave ovens, poor quality drinking water, mass vaccination programmes, electricity power lines, mobile telephones, air conditioning, aeroplanes and a thousand and one sources of physical and mental stress are all putting our bodies under pressure. Just when we need the best food we can get our food is the worst it has ever been.

In a nutshell: we need a good supply of vitamins more than ever but the quality of our food is deteriorating rapidly and we're getting fewer vitamins than before.

If you are going to take a supplement (as I now do) then in my view you should make sure that you take the best you can. There are hundreds if not thousands of products available: some will contain high levels of active ingredients and others will undoubtedly contain inactive fillers and bulking agents. If you decide to take a supplement then you should choose one which has a safe and effective level of active ingredients which are as pure as possible.

RECOMMENDED DAILY VITAMINS & MINERALS

Readers often ask me for details of the official recommended daily allowances (RDAs) for vitamins and minerals. The RDA for any particular vitamin is the minimum suggested daily intake you need to take in order to avoid health-related problems. RDAs sound a good idea but like many other things produced by committees or government departments they are, in truth, best described as guesses.

This is perhaps best illustrated by the fact that different countries have different RDAs. For example, the South African RDA for vitamin A for men is 1000 mcg. For women the figure is 800 mcg and 1300 mcg for women who are lactating. In the United Kingdom, however, the RDA for vitamin A is much lower. The figure for men is 700 mcg and for women it is 600 mcg (rising to 950 mcg when a woman is breast feeding). For some vitamins and minerals the differences are even greater. The UK RDA for potassium is 3500 mg for both men and women. In South Africa the RDA is 2000 mg for both sexes. The UK RDA for sodium is 1600 mg for men and women. In South Africa the RDA for sodium is 500 mg. In the UK the RDA for chromium is 25 mcg. In South Africa the RDA is be-tween 50 mcg and 200 mcg.

I've compared UK figures to South African figures because I happen to have both lists in front of me. But the variations exist in other countries too. For example, in the UK the RDA for phosphorus is 550 mg for both men and women but in Australia and New Zealand the RDA for phosphorus is 1000 mg for both sexes. How on earth government officials explain these differences I cannot imagine. I don't think I want to know.

Some countries don't have RDAs for vitamins and minerals for which other countries do have RDAs. The countries which do have RDAs say the figures have been established. The countries which haven't say they haven't.

All this is made even dottier by the fact that governments recommend exactly the same RDA for a man weighing 8 stones as they do for a man weighing 20 stones. Common sense suggests that the practical requirements must be very different.

Salt

We need some salt to stay healthy but most of us eat around twenty times as much salt as we need. There is salt in bread, milk, cream, cheese, butter, margarine and meat and meat products — as well as many tinned products — so avoiding salt isn't always easy.

Hundreds of scientific papers have been published by experts trying to decide just how dangerous salt can be. And the experts are divided. A few — rather vociferous — experts believe that salt is a killer. But the majority seem unconvinced as yet and admit that they don't know how bad salt is or how much salt causes real problems. (Though all experts seem generally agreed on the fact that people with high blood pressure or with a family history of high blood pressure should keep their salt intake down to a minimum.)

Although there is uncertainty about the size of the problem there is little doubt that too much salt can cause problems.

For example, salt is a serious cause of fluid retention. Avoiding or cutting down salt consumption can, therefore, help patients (such as women with the premenstrual syndrome) who suffer from symptoms created by fluid retention.

If you want to cut down your salt intake you can do so by avoiding: processed foods in general, canned foods, junk foods, crisps, salted peanuts, salted biscuits, salted butter, salted cheese, sausages and bacon. Alternative flavourings include lemon juice, parsley, garlic, horseradish and tarragon.

Seven ways to reduce your salt intake

1. Eat fewer salted snacks — such as peanuts and crisps — which tend to be heavily salted.

2. Avoid meat products — which often contain salt.

3. Avoid smoked fish and bacon — which are often salted.

4. Cook with herbs and spices rather than salt.

5. Buy spreads, sauces and pickles which are low in salt content.

6. Whenever possible use fresh vegetables rather than tinned vegetables to which extra salt has already been added.

7. Keep salt off the table.

CHAPTER TWO

SAFE DRINKING

Water

You probably don't think of water as a food but water is just as valuable as anything you eat. A massive 60% to 65% of your body is water. (The figure is even higher for a baby. Approximately 75% of a baby's weight is water.) If you didn't eat and didn't drink it would be the shortage of water which killed you first. You could survive for weeks without food but you would be dead within about seven days without water.

Your body's need for water varies according to the outside temperature. When the weather outside is hot your body will deliberately lose water as sweat to try to keep your internal body temperature low. However, even when the outside temperature is fairly low your body will lose some water in urine, in faeces and as evaporation from your skin, and will need that water replacing if you are to stay alive. You lose about two litres of water a day even when the weather isn't warm.

You don't have to drink your entire daily fluid requirements as water or as fluid, of course. Your intake of water is supplemented by the water which is present in many of the foods you eat. Some fruits and vegetables contain 90% water. To that you can add the fact that the metabolism of carbohydrates, fat and protein leads to the production of yet more water. On balance the average sized human being, living in a fairly average climate, will need at least two or three litres of fluid a day in order to satisfy his or her body's requirements, to maintain healthy kidneys and to stay in good health.

Most of us take it for granted that the water we obtain by turning on our taps will be fresh and pure. Sadly, however, there is a growing amount of evidence to show that the water most of us get when we turn on our taps isn't always quite as pure as we like to think it is.

There are four reasons why your drinking water may not be as pure as you would like:

First, much of our drinking water is contaminated with nitrates. The nitrates get into the water supplies when farmers use large quantities of artificial fertilizer. The nitrates from the fertiliser seep down into the ground and eventually find their way into the water supplies. Just what damage nitrates can do to the human body is still something of a mystery, though some people believe that they may be linked to a variety of serious disorders, including cancer.

The second problem is that many of the facilities for extracting and supplying water to the developed world are now getting rather old. Many water pipes were laid during the nineteenth century and throughout the developed world there are many people who still get their water pumped through lead pipes. Unfortunately, water that passes through lead piping has a nasty tendency to pick up quite a bit of lead before it gets to the tap. And lead in drinking water can lead to many serious problems — including damage to the brain and the central nervous system.

The third problem comes from the fact that the people whose job it is to provide us with clean water often use chemicals to disinfect, sterilise, purify or otherwise cleanse the water they are selling. Two of the substances which they are most likely to use are chlorine and aluminium sulphate and both these substances may cause problems. It is now suspected that one of the substances that is produced when chlorine mixes with the acids which naturally occur in peaty soils may cause intestinal cancer. And aluminium sulphate, used partly to help remove the acids which might otherwise interact with the chlorine to create cancer producing chemicals, and partly to take the discoloration out of peaty water, may cause problems too. The worry is that there may be a link between the drinking of aluminium rich water and the development of premature senility — in particular Alzheimer's disease. In addition to the dangers which may exist when chlorine and aluminium sulphate are added to drinking water supplies in ordinary quantities there is the extra hazard of what can happen when large quantities of a chemical are accidentally dumped into drinking water supplies — as has happened.

The fourth reason why modern drinking water supplies might be hazardous to your health involves the deliberate adding of chemicals to water in order to keep us 'healthy'. The substance most commonly added to drinking water supplies is fluoride. This is done in the hope that it will help reduce the incidence of tooth decay. The link between fluoride and tooth decay was first established at the end of the nineteenth century and there is little doubt that fluoride does help to protect the teeth by making tooth enamel — the hard outside covering of teeth — tougher and more decay resistant. When tests done on large numbers of people showed that tooth decay is slower in those parts of the country where drinking water supplies naturally contain fluoride some scientists and politicians suggested that putting fluoride into the drinking water supplies might improve the dental health of the general population. The fluoridation of water supplies began in America in 1945 and today the move towards fluoridation is spreading all over the world. Politicians are enthusiastic about using fluoride in this way because the end result is, of course, to cut health costs.

However, those who oppose fluoridation are able to put forward several arguments in their favour.

First, you do not, of course, have to add fluoride to drinking water in order to protect teeth. You can get exactly the same effect by persuading people to use fluoride toothpastes. And since many toothpastes now do contain fluoride most people already get all the fluoride they need simply by brushing their teeth.

Second, there is no doubt that putting fluoride into drinking water supplies is a potentially dangerous business. The amount of fluoride that you can put into drinking water has to be judged very accurately. To get the best effect from the fluoride you need to add around one part per million. However, if you get the sums wrong the consequences can be devastating. Just two parts of fluoride per million can cause mottling of the teeth and if the quantities are allowed to rise a little higher bone disorders and cancer may be the result. Naturally, the scientists and politicians who are keen on putting fluoride into our drinking water supplies claim that the methods used are foolproof but I think that one would have to be a fool to believe that. Many people have already been poisoned by accidental overdoses of chemicals and in 1986 the World Health Organization published a report in which concern was expressed about the incidence of dental problems caused by there being too much fluoride in public drinking water supplies. Needless to say getting unwanted, excess fluoride out of the drinking water supplies can be extremely difficult.

To all this we must add the fact that since drinking water supplies already contain a number of chemicals — some of which occur naturally in the supplies, nitrates which accumulate because of the use of fertilizers, chlorine and aluminium sulphate which are added deliberately and lead or copper from the pipes which are used to supply the water to our homes — adding fluoride to the mixture may increase the risk of a dangerous interaction between the various chemicals in the water. Whenever chemicals exist in solution together there are chemical reactions. I don't think anyone really knows what the consequences are of putting all these chemicals into our drinking water.

The fourth anti fluoridation argument is that a growing number of people seem to be allergic to the chemicals which are being put into our drinking water. Many people are allergic to fluoride and cannot drink fluoridated drinking water.

Finally, I am particularly worried by the fact that as the pro fluoridation argument is won in more and more parts of the world, scientists and politicians are suggesting putting other chemicals into the drinking water supplies. One scientist has, for example, already suggested that drinking water should have antibiotics added to it (to reduce the incidence of infection and so to reduce health costs). Another has recommended that tranquillisers be added to drinking water supplies (in order to calm down the voters and allow the politicians to get on with running the world the way they want to run it). A third suggestion has been that contraceptives be added to the drinking water in order to reduce the birth rate.

THE CONTAMINATION OF OUR DRINKING WATER

Back in 1982 — in a column I was writing in a medical journal — I raised the question of whether or not public drinking water supplies could be polluted with female hormone residues which might affect the development of male babies.

I tried to get television and radio journalists to take up the problem. And I tried to interest politicians in the topic too. But although many were horrified by the idea all quickly decided that it was far too controversial a subject.

'It'll frighten people far too much!' was the common view.

However, it wasn't just the possibility of female hormones — residues from the contraceptive pill — which might be causing problems which worried me. At the time when I first wrote about this subject I was so alarmed by what I had discovered that I spent over a year doing research before I wrote the article and my fear was built on several pieces of information.

* Fact one: More and more people are taking increasingly powerful medicinal drugs such as antibiotics, painkillers, tranquillisers, sleeping tablets, hormones (particularly those in the contraceptive pill) and steroids. Huge numbers of people take drugs every day. Not many people go through a whole year without taking at least one course of tablets. Half of the population will take a prescribed medicine today (and tomorrow and the day after that). And on top of the prescribed drugs there are all the non prescription drugs that are taken — pills bought over the chemists counter and taken day in and day out.

* Fact two: Many drugs are excreted in the urine when the body has finished with them. For example, up to 75% of a dose of a tranquilliser may be excreted in the urine. With other drugs the figure may be as high as 90%. Some drugs which are degraded can chemically react with the environment and become active again.

* Fact three: After going through standard purification procedures waste water is often discharged into fresh water rivers.

Fact four. Drinking water supplies are often taken from fresh water rivers — the same rivers into which the waste water has been discharged.

* Fact five: Water purification programmes were designed many years ago — before doctors started prescribing vast quantities of drugs for millions of patients and before the problem of removing drug residues had been thought of.

I felt that even someone with a modest IQ should be able to see where all this was leading.

It seemed clear to me that anyone who turned on a tap and made a cup of tea could be getting a cocktail containing leftover chemicals from other people's tranquillisers, sleeping pills, antibiotics, contraceptive pills, heart drugs, anti-arthritis pills and so on.

Back in 1982 I wrote that: 'with an increasing number of people taking drugs there must be a risk that the drinking water supplies will eventually become contaminated so heavily that people using ordinary drinking water will effectively be taking drugs. Or have we already reached that point: and are people who drink water in certain areas of the country already passively involved in daily drug taking?'

Back in 1982 no one seemed to know the answer to that frightening question.

And today I still don't know the answer.

Does anyone?

Are you an involuntary drug taker? Could you be addicted to any of the drug residues which might be in your drinking water? Could you be taking regular supplies of bits and pieces of other people's antibiotics? Are you taking contraceptive hormone leftovers? Could these drug residues be affecting your fertility? Could drug residues affect the health of any unborn children?

No one in government seems concerned by these questions.

I think they should be.

It may soon be too late, for evidence is already appearing to suggest that my original fears were accurate.

A report published in 1999 by the Environmental Agency in the UK reports that 57% of the roach in one river had changed sex. Chemicals in treated sewage and factory waste were blamed for upsetting natural fish hormones. The researchers found that the fish were more likely to be affected when they spent time close to a sewage outlet. They also found that fish who lived upstream (away from the sewage outlet) were much less likely to be affected. Apparently, the chemicals in sewage which are most likely to affect fish are female hormones such as oestrogens.

Strangely, some scientists still seem puzzled about the source of the female hormones. (Since the average scientist seems to have the IQ of a dead tree one should not, I suppose, be too surprised by this.)

While they were studying lake water for pesticide contamination Swiss chemists were surprised to find that the lake was polluted with clofibric acid — a drug which is used to lower blood cholesterol levels. The possibility that this could have been caused by industrial spillage was ruled out when it was established that clofibric acid is not manufactured in Switzerland. When the chemists checked other lakes and rivers they found low concentrates of the drug everywhere.

When researchers in Germany started looking for clofibric acid they found the drug in all sorts of water supplies — including tap water.

Intrigued, the researchers looked harder.

And they found lipid-lowering drugs, analgesics (including diclofenac and ibuprofen), beta blocker heart drugs, antibiotics, chemotherapy drugs and hormones. They found all these drugs in water bodies and in drinking water. And they found that the concentrations were highest in heavily populated areas. Once they had ruled out industrial spillage the researchers realised that the drugs had come from human body wastes. Exactly what I had predicted in 1982.

The chances are that no one knows what drugs can be found in your drinking water. Why? Because no one is looking. Most governments do not monitor water supplies to see if they contain drug residues. Nor do they require anyone else to do this.

But there seems little doubt that drinking water is now heavily contaminated with drug residues. And the long term effect of all this is difficult to estimate. Minute amounts of antibiotics in drinking water can affect bacteria in many different ways. They can surely have a dramatic effect on the development of antibiotic-resistant organisms.

There is not yet any evidence showing a clear link between water pollution and problems (such as fertility) affecting human beings. But the absence of any such evidence may possibly be a result of the fact that as far as I know no one has yet done any research into this issue. The research would be extremely simple to do and wouldn't cost very much. Scientists would simply count the number of people with fertility problems (or some other specific disorder) who had drunk re-circulated water and then compare that figure with the incidence of fertility problems among people who had drunk fresh spring or borehole water. But who would want to do such research? Certainly not the water companies.

How are the drugs in your drinking water affecting your health? Is your daily cocktail of tranquillisers, antibiotics, hormones, steroids, chemotherapy drugs, heart drugs, pain killers and so on making you ill? How do all these drugs interact? Are they likely to be at least partly responsible for the way the incidence of cancer is increasing? Are they affecting your immune system?

No one knows.

And no one in authority seems to want to know.

Maybe they are frightened to discover the truth.

Meanwhile, politicians around the world now drink spring water, at taxpayers' expense, which is bottled at source before it has too much chance of becoming contaminated.

DON'T DRINK UNFILTERED TAP WATER

You should drink six to eight decent sized glasses of water a day. Fizzy drinks and caffeinated teas and coffees don't count. Nor do alcoholic drinks. Caffeine and alcohol are diuretics which cause the body to lose water. If you can't bear the idea of drinking that much water look for drinks that contain no alcohol, no caffeine and no sugar or sodium. Herbal, fruit or mint teas are fine as are decaffeinated drinks. Alternatively, you can try drinking pure fruit juice diluted with water.

If you want to drink plain water I suggest you avoid tap water. In most countries governments make sure that tap water is regulated and undergoes rigorous tests which means, I'm afraid, that it is pretty much undrinkable and best used for doing the washing up unless you use a filter. Bottled drinking water isn't necessarily pure. Some 'spring water' has been purified or chemically treated while the stuff sold as 'table water' may be nothing more than filtered tap water.

The best bet is probably 'natural mineral water' which comes from a protected, pure, unadulterated source and should not have been treated or tampered with. Natural mineral water may contain some bacteria (though not usually enough to do you any harm) and so you shouldn't keep bottled natural mineral water lying around once the bottle has been opened.

HOW TO PROTECT YOURSELF FROM 'POLLUTED' DRINKING WATER

1. If you suffer from any bizarre or otherwise inexplicable symptoms consider the possibility that your drinking water may be polluted. And it could be the water which is making you ill. This is particularly likely to be the case if you have acquired any new and unusual health problems after recently moving house.

2. Small babies should be breast fed for as long as possible — ideally for up to twelve months. Breast feeding a baby reduces the risk of the baby being poisoned by polluted water or milk (though it does not reduce the risk to nil since drugs are excreted in breast milk).

3. If you suspect that any symptoms which you have could be caused by drinking water obtained from a tap try drinking bottled water instead to see if your symptoms disappear.

4. If you live in the country and you can do so then you may be better off obtaining your water from a private water supply. But do make sure that you get your water tested before drinking it.

5. Even if you obtain your water from a commercial company or government owned concern you would be wise to have it tested — as it comes out of the tap.

6. You can buy table top small filters which remove many contaminants from drinking water. If you buy and use one of these devices make sure that you follow the manufacturer's instructions.

7. If you suspect that your drinking water supplies are of poor quality make your protests heard by your political representatives. Things will never change if you do not protest.

Alcohol and Alcoholism

The liver isn't the only organ damaged by too much drinking of alcohol. Stomach ulcers, muscle wastage, cancer and brain disease all occur in alcoholics. The incidence of alcoholism is going up fast as more women drink to excess. Early physical symptoms include hand tremor, indigestion, poor appetite, impotence, fits, blackouts, memory lapses and frequent accidents. Anxiety, depression and restlessness at night are also common. Most alcoholics do enormous damage to those around them as they lie, steal and break the law. Half of road deaths are caused by alcoholics. Alcoholism is an addiction but it can be treated.

Alcohol: weekly drink limit

For men the weekly limit is 21 units spread throughout the week. For women the weekly limit is 14 units spread throughout the week.

How much alcohol is there in your drink?

 1 pint of ordinary strength beer or lager contains 2 units

 1 pint export beer or lager contains 2.5 units

 1 pint strong beer or lager contains 4 units

 1 pint extra strong beer or lager contains 5 units

 1 pint cider contains 3 units

 1 pint strong cider contains 4 units

 1 average glass of wine contains 1 unit (pub measure)

 1 average glass of sherry, port or vermouth contains 1 unit (pub measure)

 1 average glass of liqueur contains 1 unit (pub measure)

1 single of spirits contains 1 unit (pub measure)

Caffeine

Are you a caffeine addict?
Do you regularly suffer from headaches, indigestion or palpitations?
Do you get edgy, irritable and nervous?
Do you ever feel tired and washed out?
Do you have difficulty in getting to sleep at night?

If you have answered 'yes' to any of these questions then there could be a simple explanation. For if, in addition to suffering from any of the symptoms I have listed, you also drink more than three or four cups of coffee and/or tea a day then you could be a caffeine addict.

And the symptoms you are getting could be a result of your addiction.

Caffeine is one of the most powerful stimulants in the world. The largest pharmacology textbook in my library devotes more space to caffeine than it does to cannabis or amphetamine.

Taken regularly or in high doses caffeine will send your blood pressure sky high and make your heart beat faster. Caffeine causes trouble when the daily intake exceeds 250 mg and since a cup of tea contains between 50 and 100 mg of caffeine and a cup of coffee contains between 75 and 150 mg of caffeine just three or four cups a day is all you need to produce symptoms.

But if you are thinking of cutting down do take care. If you cut down too quickly then you could get withdrawal symptoms such as headaches, depression, anxiety and irritability. To avoid these problems cut down slowly either by drinking fewer cups or by taking your tea or coffee weaker. An alternative long-term solution is to try decaffeinated coffee or herbal tea.

TOO MUCH COFFEE OR TEA MAY INCREASE YOUR CHANCES OF DEVELOPING HEART DISEASE

Heart disease is the biggest killer in all Western style countries.

And, although not all experts agree, there is plenty of research and expert material available to show that there is a link between caffeine-rich drinks and heart disease.

* In a study of 1,130 medical students, reported in the *New England Journal of Medicine,* it was reported that 'the relative risks of coronary heart disease for men drinking five or more cups of coffee a day, as compared to non-drinkers, were approx. 2.49'.

* Caffeine is a powerful stimulant affecting the heart and its arteries as well as kidneys, lungs, brain and central nervous system.

* Large amounts of coffee can cause a temporary increase in heart rate and blood pressure. If there is any tendency to extra heart beats or palpitations then the caffeine in coffee can make this worse.

* Coffee may trigger odd (ectopic) beats. If you are troubled by odd heart beats it might be better to cut down your coffee intake.

* Excessive coffee drinking (5 or 6 cups or more per day) is likely to be associated with a raised level of blood cholesterol.

* In a study which involved 1,596 men and women it was shown that there is a significant association between coffee consumption and blood cholesterol levels.

Coffee isn't just a possible cause of heart symptoms.

Despite its wide availability caffeine (the active substance in the 5 million tonnes of coffee sold annually) is a remarkably powerful stimulant; it stimulates the brain and nervous system; it increases the effect of acid on the stomach and it stimulates the kidneys.

Researchers have claimed that too much caffeine can lead to muscle tremors, insomnia, anxiety, depression, headaches, indigestion, palpitations, bowel problems and personality changes.

Numerous scientific research studies have shown that caffeine containing beverages can be dangerous in other ways. After a critical assessment of a large number of experimental and epidemiological studies the International Agency for Research on Cancer recently concluded that coffee may cause bladder cancer while drinking tea may increase the risk of oesophageal cancer.

Cow's Milk

Milk has a tremendous reputation as a healthy food. The consumption of milk has been rising steadily for decades. But that reputation is hardly deserved.

Here are three health reasons why I don't drink cow's milk — a drink which is really only suitable for calves. (I also object to the way cows are 'farmed' but that is a moral question.)

1. Milk contains fat which can clog up your arteries and increase your chances of having a heart attack. Amazingly most people still seem to drink milk which contains lots of fat — instead of the much healthier, low fat skimmed and semi-skimmed varieties.

2. Cow's milk can cause allergies and digestive troubles. Eczema, asthma, migraine, irritable bowel syndrome and sinus problems are just five of the common disorders believed to be associated with milk drinking.

3. Most worrying is the fact that some farmers give their cows hormones to increase their milk yield. What effect will these hormones have on you and your family? I don't know. And I don't think anyone else knows either.

Soya Milk

Soya milk — made by washing, soaking and grinding soya beans and then mixing them with boiling water — is an excellent alternative to cow's milk.

Soya milk (and soya yoghurt and ice cream are also available) contains no cholesterol, little sugar and plenty of protein. The fats in soya milk are of the polyunsaturated kind (in cow's milk the fats are saturated). Soya milk can easily be used as a replacement for cow's milk and although you would be able to tell the difference if you drank the two straight from a glass you probably won't be able to tell the difference if you used the soya milk on cereal or in cooking.

CHAPTER THREE

HOW HEALTHY ARE YOUR EATING HABITS?

You may think your diet is healthy. But let's find out!

Answer the questions in this simple quiz to find out exactly how healthy your eating habits really are.

1. Which sort of bread do you usually buy?
a) white
b) wholemeal

2. Do you eat an average of one piece of fresh fruit?
a) every day?
b) most days?
c) occasionally?
d) rarely?
e) never?

3. Where do you get most of your vegetables from?
a) own garden (or friend's garden)
b) fresh from the greengrocer
c) ready packaged or tinned

4. What sort of milk do you buy?
a) extra cream
b) ordinary
c) skimmed
d) semi-skimmed
e) soya

6. When you eat meals do you
a) tend to eat in a rush?
b) usually make sure that you allow yourself enough time?

7. Do you eat sweets or chocolates
a) every day or nearly every day?
b) most days of the week?
c) occasionally?
d) rarely?
e) never?

8. Do you
a) eat unlimited amounts of sugar?
b) make a conscious effort to control the amount of sugar you eat?
c) keep the amount of sugar you eat to a minimum?

9. Do you
a) eat meat every day?
b) eat meat most days?
c) eat meat occasionally?
d) eat meat rarely?
e) never eat meat at all?

10. When buying pasta or rice do you
a) usually buy the white variety?
b) usually buy the wholemeal or brown variety?

11. How many times a week do you eat beans, peas or lentils?
a) at least once a day

b) most days

c) occasionally

d) rarely

e) never

12. How often do you eat cakes, buns, pastries or biscuits?

a) at least once a day

b) most days

c) occasionally

d) rarely

e) never

13. Do you usually use?

a) butter

b) a low fat spread

c) a very low fat spread

14. Do you make a conscious effort to limit your fat intake?

a) yes

b) no

15. Do you make a conscious effort to keep your fibre intake high?

a) yes

b) no

NOW CHECK YOUR SCORE

1. a) 0 b) 5

2. a) 5 b) 4 c) 3 d) 2 e) 1

3. a) 5 b) 3 c) 1

4. a) 0 b) 1 c) 3 d) 5 e) 5

5. a) 3 b) 0
6. a) 0 b) 3
7. a) 0 b) 1 c) 2 d) 3 e) 5
8. a) 0 b) 3 c) 5
9. a) 0 b) 1 c) 2 d) 3 e) 5
10. a) 0 b) 3
11. a) 5 b) 4 c) 3 d) 1 e) 0
12. a) 0 b) 1 c) 3 d) 4 e) 5
13. a) 0 b) 3 c) 5
14. a) 5 b) 0
15. a) 5 b) 0

If you scored 60 or more then your diet is a healthy one.

If you scored less than 60 you could improve your health noticeably by taking more care with your diet.

Do you put your convenience before your health?
The shops are full of 'convenience' foods these days: packets and tins of prepared food which require no kitchen skills but which provide a ready to eat meal in just a few minutes. Sadly, these 'convenience' foods are often low in fibre, vitamins and minerals and high in fat. If you're living on a diet of convenience foods you could be endangering your health.

CHAPTER FOUR

FOOD ADDITIVES

Food manufacturers use flavourings, preservatives and colourings to restore or improve the taste, texture or colour of the foods they sell. Altogether they use several thousand different additives and in recent years there has been a considerable amount of discussion about the safety of these substances. Since the average consumer eats around 5.5lb (2.5kg) of additives every year the problem clearly *could* be a massive one. Additives enable manufacturers to debase foods in order to increase their own profits.

No one has the foggiest idea how safe food additives are but I honestly don't think anyone in power gives a stuff about this. I have in front of me a booklet which was published by a government agency. In this booklet the government sternly warns that 'ham and bacon couldn't be sold without the preservative that also gives them their pink colour' and claims that 'scientists and doctors who check safety evidence for the government are satisfied the use of these additives is safe'.

Feel better?

No, I thought not.

And you are right to be sceptical.

When bravely explaining the fact that flavourings are not controlled as tightly as other additives the same booklet boldly admits that this is because there are over 3,000 flavourings in use, in many different combinations.

So, there you have it.

One official reason for not controlling flavourings tightly is that there are too many of them to control properly.

My advice is to consume as few additives as you possibly can. Try to eat fresh food whenever possible and avoid buying pre-packed foods that are stuffed with chemicals.

Food Additives And Cancer

Food ingredients which may cause cancer in humans include the polycyclic aromatic hydrocarbons (the concentration of which is increased by burning, overcooking or barbecuing); the nitrosamines (which may be formed by a reaction between substances normally present in food and the nitrates or nitrates which are added to fish, sausages, bacon, ham cheese etc. in order to stop the food from 'spoiling') and moulds which grow on foods which are normally free of carcinogens and then produce toxic substances called mycotoxins (the fungus called ergot which grows on rye and causes womb contractions in healthy women has been used as a prescription drug and is the substance from which LSD was created). The aflatoxins, which grow on peanuts, are among the most powerful of all carcinogenic substances.

It is, however, the artificial additives which are added to food as preservatives, colourings and flavourings which worry consumers most. Theoretically, chemicals which are added to food are subjected to extensive testing to make sure that they are not dangerous. But the value of many of the tests which are performed must be in question. 'The interpretation of studies which appear to show the potential for tumour formation in animals is becoming increasingly difficult,' said the British Medical Association in its book *The BMA Guide to Living With Risk* (published by Penguin in 1990). 'Some testing procedures are very tightly standardised, but have little relationship to the real world or to use by humans. Other tests are more flexible but difficult to relate one to the other. Indeed, a great deal more needs to be known about the induction of cancer in animals by chemicals before the findings can be confidently related to man.' (One wonders why scientists don't just forget about the animal experiments completely and concentrate on human studies. They could do preliminary toxicity and carcinogenicity tests on human tissue and organ samples and then study limits cohort samples in order to investigate the long-term carcinogenicity in humans.)

'Chemicals that cause cancer are a diverse group which act in different ways,' says the British Medical Association. 'To classify all of them for the purpose of regulation as 'carcinogens' is not very logical today, because we really do not know what some of the laboratory findings in animals actually mean, and the mechanism of action of chemical carcinogens in biochemical terms is very unclear. Some of the testing defies common sense. If a chemical is administered to a rat in relatively enormous amounts there will be absolutely inevitable changes in that part of the diet which remains and is acceptable to that unfortunate animal, its metabolism is bound to be altered, and these changes may or may not have as much influence on the animal's illness as the chemical itself.'

'In summary, then,' said the BMA, 'carcinogens in food are more likely to be there 'naturally' or as a result of traditional preservation methods than by the addition of synthetic chemicals. The significance to human beings of very tiny amounts of carcinogens (as assessed through animal experimentation) is unknown. It would be hard to live on a diet which contained no substances which at some time had been shown by laboratory or animal tests to have carcinogenic properties.' The British Medical Association has also pointed out that: 'if salt and sugar were being tested as potential food additives today, and if judgement of acceptability was to be based purely on the laboratory and animal testing, it is unlikely that either would be permitted for use in food.'

In my view food additives are potential hazards. They are best avoided as much as possible and this is best done by eating as much fresh food as possible.

The types of additives

1. Flavourings

Flavourings are sometimes added to give added or extra or enhanced flavour to a product and they are sometimes used to give an entirely different flavour to a rather bland product or to a product which has an unpleasant taste. Monosodium glutamate is often used to stimulate the taste buds and increase the sensation of flavour — despite the fact that it can cause severe headaches. Manufacturers who use flavourings well can make just about anything — including a ground up telephone directory — taste good.

2. Colourings

Colourings are often added to make food look more like the pictures on the packaging. Without colourings, many prepackaged foods would probably look dull and unappetising.

Sometimes colourings are deliberately used to deceive customers. For example, companies making meat products will use a red dye to disguise the fat and other non-meat ingredients in pies and sausages. Sometimes there isn't much logic in the way in which colourings are used. For example, custard consists mainly of corn starch flavoured with vanilla but contains a dye to make it look yellow. This is done because when custard was first introduced the customers were persuaded that the product was made from eggs. Not many people still believe that custard has anything at all to do with eggs but the yellow colour has become 'normal' and so the dye is invariably added to the mix.

3. *Preservatives*

Preservatives are used to stop micro organisms developing — and to slow down the rate at which products go bad. Amazingly, some preservatives are included to stop the colourings fading or the flavourings going 'off'.

4. *Emulsifiers*

Emulsifiers are used so that water can be included in a product. There are two reasons to do this. First, water helps to give a product a smooth, firm texture. Second, water is cheap and helps to increase the weight of a product without adding to its cost. Food manufacturers often use water and emulsifiers to increase the weight of meat products.

5. *Stabilizers*

Stabilisers are used, often in conjunction with emulsifiers, to stop water and fat separating and, therefore, to improve the smoothness and creaminess of a food.

6. *Acids*

Are used to help preserve food and to give it a sharper taste.

7. *Anti-caking agent*

Added to stop food being lumpy.

8. *Bulking agent*

Added to make you feel fuller and more satisfied after a meal.

9. *Sweeteners*

Added to make a food taste sweeter.

10. *Thickeners*

Are used to make food thicker and to improve its consistency.

11. *Glazing agents*

May help to preserve food but also used to give food a shiny look.

12. *The rest*

Many of the available food additives are used to make foods easier to process or pack. Some are included to make a product easier to spread or to improve its consistency in other ways. Manufacturers sometimes add anti splattering agents to stop oil splashing out when wet chips are added. Additives can, if used properly, enable a manufacturer to make a food look or taste like virtually anything. Because meat tends to be expensive the most common use of additives is in the preparation of meat products (which sometimes contain very little genuine meat).

THE HARM ADDITIVES CAN DO

Additives included in food can kill vitamins and cause a massive variety of symptoms and diseases including: asthma, eczema, dermatitis, migraine, hyperactivity in children, dizziness, kidney problems, diarrhoea, fits, palpitations, stomach pains, intestinal disorders and allergy problems.

Many of the most commonly used additives have never been tested to see if they are safe for human consumption. Those working in the food industry excuse this bizarre fact by pointing out that there are several thousand additives in use and that testing procedures are lengthy, expensive and time consuming. I doubt if many consumers will take more comfort from this.

I have heard some food company representatives defending the use of food additives by saying that only 1 in a 1000 people are likely to be adversely affected by a particular additive. I don't find that particularly comforting for 1 in 1000 is not good odds. If

1,000,000 eat a particular food then a 1 in 1,000 risk means that 1,000 people are going to be made ill by it.

I am also worried by the fact that many different additives are often used together. It is widely acknowledged that chemicals often interact. If you include two different chemical substances in one product then there is a real risk that the two will combine and produce something quite different. Modern foods contain so many different additives that it is quite easy to eat a meal which contains fifty different chemicals.

No one knows what all those additives are likely to do to your health. No one knows what long term side effects may be building up. No one knows how those additives are likely to interact with one another.

Five tips to help you limit the number of additives you consume

1. In order to minimise your consumption of food additives I suggest that you try to buy as many fresh foods as you possibly can.

2. When you do buy processed or packaged foods try to buy products with a short list of additives. It is well worth remembering that the substance named first on the packet is usually the one that appears in the largest quantity inside the packet — other products should appear on the list in decreas-ing order of quantity.

3. Grow as much of your own food as you possibly can. Even if you only have a small garden you may be able to grow many of your own vegetables.

4. If you (or anyone in your family) develop new or unusual symptoms after eating a new product try to avoid that product in future.

5. Become a cynic when reading food advertisements and food labels. Over the last few years the food industry has managed to devalue the word 'natural' so that it has become virtually meaningless. For example, the phrase 'only natural ingredients' is sometimes used to describe foods which are stuffed with additives if those additives are chemicals that occur naturally, or synthetic versions of chemicals which occur naturally.

E Numbers to Avoid

In countries within the European Community some food additives are given E numbers so that consumers can tell what they are buying. The E numbers contained within a food are usually listed on the packet or tin.

Though this list of potentially troublesome additives is by no means exhaustive here are ten E numbers which I think you should try to avoid whenever possible. Make a copy of this list when you go shopping. Try to find products that do not include any of these additives. And try to avoid *all* additives as much as you can.

1. E102 (tartrazine)
2. E 110 (sunset yellow)
3. E123 (amaranth)
4. E127 (erythrosine)
5. E132 (indigo carmine)
6. E153 (carbon black)
7. E173 (aluminium)

8. E210 (benzoic acid)

9. E222 (sodium hydrogen sulphite)

10. E321 (butylated hydroxytoluene)

CHAPTER FIVE

HOW MUCH DO YOU KNOW ABOUT FOOD SAFETY?

Food poisoning is a major problem — frequently caused by carelessness and bad habits in the kitchen. Do this quiz to find out how much you know about preparing food the healthy way.

1. Which of these foods is safest to eat in the street?

a) bananas

b) oranges

c) hot dog

d) hamburger

2. You have got raw meat defrosting in the fridge. Where should you store it?

a) on the top shelf

b) it doesn't matter

c) on the bottom shelf

3. Which of these is true?

a) you should store cooked food away from uncooked food

b) you should always cover up food that has been prepared

c) raw meat is safer to eat than cooked meat

4. Which of these infections is most dangerous?

a) botulism

b) salmonella

c) listeria

5. Is it safe to cook meat taken straight out of the freezer?

a) yes

b) no

6. Which of these creatures carry infection?

a) flies

b) mice

c) rats

7. After preparing an uncooked chicken you should always:

a) wash the knife and cutting board thoroughly

b) wash your hands well

c) dispose of the waste carefully and quickly

8. Why shouldn't you put hot food into the fridge?

a) because it will develop salmonella

b) because it will heat up other food stored in the fridge and increase the chance of that food developing an infection

c) because it will go bad more rapidly

9. The symptoms of food poisoning can occur up to how long after eating infected food?

a) 4 hours

b) 24 hours

c) 5 days

10. Which type of food should be avoided by pregnant women?

a) apples

b) soft cheeses

c) fish

11. How cold should your fridge be?

a) between 3 degrees Centigrade and freezing

b) 32 degrees Centigrade below zero

c) 12 degrees Centigrade or below

12. Which of these symptoms can suggest food poisoning?

a) headache

b) vomiting

c) diarrhoea

13. Why is listeria dangerous to pregnant women?

a) it can cause a miscarriage

b) it may affect the unborn baby

c) it can affect the production of breast milk

14. Which of these is a common cause of salmonella poisoning?

a) poultry

b) fruit

c) milk

15. How hot should food get to make sure that it is cooked properly?

a) 70 degrees Centigrade

b) 50 degrees Centigrade

c) 30 degrees Centigrade

NOW CHECK YOUR SCORE

1. a) 2 points b) 2 points c) 0 points d) 0 points

Bananas and oranges — which come wrapped in their own disposable wrapping — are the safest 'street' foods you can buy.

2. a) 0 points b) 0 points c) 2 points
You should store meat on the bottom shelf so that any blood dripping from it doesn't contaminate other food.

3. a) 2 points b) 2 points c) 0 points
Raw meat is one of the most dangerous types of food you can eat.

4. a) 2 points b) 0 points c) 0 points
Botulism is by far the most dangerous bug you are likely to come in contact with through eating food.

5. a) 0 points b) 2 points
Meat needs to be thawed properly before being cooked — otherwise there is a risk that the meat in the centre will not be cooked properly when you eat it.

6. a) 1 point b) 1 point c) 1 point
All these creatures can, of course, carry infection.

7. a) 1 point b) 1 point c) 1 point
You should do all these things.

8. a) 0 points b) 2 points c) 0 points
If you put hot food into the fridge it will increase the temperature inside the fridge and other food stored there may rise in temperature to a dangerous level.

9. a) 0 points b) 0 points c) 2 points
Food poisoning can occur up to 5 days after eating infected food.

10. a) 0 points b) 2 points c) 0 points
Pregnant women should avoid soft cheeses — and other foods made with unpasteurised milk. These are likely to contain listeria.

11. a) 2 points b) 0 points c) 0 points
You should keep your refrigerator between freezing and 3 degrees Centigrade in order to keep bugs at bay.

12. a) 2 points b) 2 points c) 2 points
Each of these symptoms can be produced by food poisoning.

13. a) 1 point b) 1 point c) 0 points
Listeria can cause miscarriages and can affect an unborn baby.

14. a) 2 points b) 0 points c) 0 points
Poultry is a common cause of salmonella poisoning.

15. a) 2 points b) 0 points c) 0 points
Food should be cooked at 70 degrees Centigrade or above to make sure that bugs are destroyed.

If you scored less than 30 points you should read this section of the book very carefully.

Food Poisoning

Stomach pain, vomiting and diarrhoea are the classic symptoms of food poisoning — a syndrome caused by eating contaminated food.

If several members of the same family all develop these symptoms after eating the same meal then food poisoning has to be suspected. Some types of food poisoning begin within hours — even minutes — while others may take days to develop.

If you think you might have contracted food poisoning: rest, avoid solids, drink plenty of fluids and contact your doctor for advice.

Botulism

Botulism is one of the most deadly and horrifying diseases known to man. The toxin produced by the Clostridium botulinum bacteria — probably the most poisonous substance in the world — is so deadly that one small drop can kill 50,000 people.

Unlike most types of food poisoning botulism affects the nervous system rather than the stomach. There may be some nausea and vomiting a few hours after eating contaminated food but the first real symptoms usually start fairly suddenly 18 to 36 hours after the food was eaten.

The faster symptoms start the more serious the disease is likely to be.

The symptoms to watch out for are (in the order in which they may appear):
* tiredness
* dizziness
* blurred or double vision
* dry mouth
* difficulty in swallowing
* slurred speech
* breathing difficulties
* general weakness of arms and legs.

As the disease spreads through the body so the paralysis spreads and becomes gradually more and more severe. One of the most terrifying aspects of the disease is that patients remain fully alert as the paralysis spreads. Because there is no effect on mental skills patients remain fully aware of what is happening to them. Doctors usually have to inject calming drugs in order to help prevent understandable panic.

Botulism is so deadly that it kills up to 70% of the patients who get it if they are not treated quickly and properly.

Since the chest muscles which control breathing are often affected patients will frequently need to be put onto a respirator and looked after in an intensive care unit.

A tracheotomy — in which a life saving tube is inserted into the patient's windpipe — is often essential as the poison spreads.

Anti-toxins — to combat the poison — are usually given not only to people who have the disease but also to those who have eaten the poisonous food but have not yet shown signs of the disease — though this must be done within hours.

The bacteria which cause botulism cannot survive in the presence of oxygen and normally live buried in the soil — which is how they get into food. Heat and sterilisation techniques usually prevent botulism. It is usually home preserved foods that are usually the cause of the disease — vegetables, fruits and meats can all cause it.

Here are three additional reasons why botulism needs to be taken seriously:

1. The poison produced by the botulism organism is probably the most deadly substance in the world. No one is immune. One yoghurt carton full of botulism poison could wipe out an entire nation.

2. Botulism is so rare that relatively little of the potentially life-saving botulism anti-toxin is kept in stock.

3. Victims of botulism poisoning usually need to be treated in special intensive care units — and many need to be kept alive on life support machines and ventilators until the paralysis produced by the poison wears off. But there are never many spare intensive care unit beds available.

Salmonella

Salmonella infections are responsible for many types of food poisoning and for the disease 'typhoid fever'. Infection of hens' eggs with salmonella is believed to be widespread.

The symptoms of salmonella food poisoning usually include headache, nausea, abdominal pain, diarrhoea and a feeling of weakness. Symptoms generally last only for a few days. Patients are usually advised to avoid solid food for the first twenty four hours of their illness but to drink plenty of fluids.

Salmonella organisms are particularly likely to be present in raw or lightly-cooked foods.

20 Point Plan For Reducing Your Chances of Developing Food Poisoning

The widespread use of preservatives to keep food in good condition has not stopped the incidence of food poisoning. The majority of food borne infections are transmitted via meat and meat products. Here are twenty tips to help you reduce your chances of acquiring a food transmitted infection.

1. Make sure that you always check the sell by date on any packaged food you buy. Sell by dates are important — and they are there for a reason. If you buy food that has gone past its sell by date you may save money but you could be putting yourself at risk.

2. Don't ever buy tins which are rusty or bulging or badly damaged (the food inside might be contaminated) and do not buy packets of food if the packet is damaged or torn.

3. When choosing food from a freezer in a store make sure that the freezer is working (i.e. is cold) and that the food is cold when you take it out. Make sure that you put the food into your freezer as soon as possible and if possible transport it home in a 'cool bag'. If you drive around with cold food in your car and it defrosts then the growth of bacteria will be encouraged.

4. Don't ever buy anything from a food shop which looks dirty. And don't buy anything from a food shop assistant who has dirty hands. The reason for this is simple: if the manager of the shop can't be bothered to ensure that the shop and his staff are clean then the chances are that he is not too fussy about food hygiene either.

5. When you are buying eggs don't buy eggs which are cracked (it is obviously easier for the egg inside to become infected if the shell is cracked). And try to buy eggs which have been laid by free range chickens rather than chickens kept in tiny cages. (Apart from the moral reasons chickens which are al-lowed to roam around are likely to be healthier than chickens kept in cages.)

6. When you store food in the fridge try to keep different types of food apart from one another in order to reduce the risk of cross contamination. Make sure that you put meat — and any other foods which are defrosting — on a plate at the bottom of the fridge so that drips won't fall onto other foods. Always keep meat (a high risk source of infection) well away from other foods.

7. Do make sure that your fridge is kept cold enough. The temperature inside your fridge should be below 3 degrees Centigrade. If your fridge is too warm then the food in it will spoil so make sure that you check the thermostat if necessary. Your fridge will work more efficiently if you defrost it regularly.

8. Never ever re-freeze food which has been frozen and already thawed. Thawing increases the number of bacteria and refreezing food increases your chances of being infected.

9. If you eat meat it is vitally important that you make sure that it is completely thawed before you start to cook it. If you don't do this then there is a risk that the middle of the meat will still be frozen when you start to cook it. If this happens then when you think all the meat is cooked the centre will still be uncooked — and probably full of bugs. It is particularly important that poultry is properly thawed before being cooked.

10. Once an item of food has been thawed make sure that you use it quickly. Do not leave it sitting around in the kitchen — if you do then micro organisms will be given a chance to multiply.

11. Always wash vegetables and fruit thoroughly in running water before using them. You should, of course, even wash food which you have grown yourself since some bugs can be carried in the soil.

12. Take care to ensure that all the worktops and equipment in your kitchen are kept scrupulously clean. Wash with soapy water; rinse afterwards in clean water and dry surfaces and utensils carefully with a clean cloth. Dirty cloths are one of the commonest causes of infection in the kitchen. It is better to let dishes and utensils drip and drain if possible. Do not use old or dirty dish cloths and change towels regularly (disposable paper towels are best because they keep the risk of cross infection to an absolute minimum).

13. Make sure that you wash your hands thoroughly before you start preparing any food — and after any interruption. If you have any infected or open wound make sure that you always wear a proper plaster or bandage (both to protect the food you are handling and yourself). Always wash your hands thoroughly after handling meat of any kind.

14. When food has been cooked you should, if possible, eat it quickly. If food which has been cooked is allowed to cool then any bugs in it will multiply. The risk increases with the length of time that cooked food is left. Cooked food which is stored should be kept cold in the fridge or hot in the oven. If you intend to eat foods which have been previously cooked make sure that you thoroughly reheat them. When reheating food it is essential that all parts of the food reach a temperature of at least 70 degrees Centigrade.

15. The best way to kill the bugs in meat, poultry or fish is to ensure that you cook the food properly. Avoid dishes which include raw meat, raw poultry or raw fish.

16. Anyone pregnant, elderly or frail should avoid soft cheeses (such as Brie and Camembert) and blue veined cheeses since these can be contaminated with listeria bacteria.

17. Don't eat raw eggs or dishes prepared with raw eggs (if you do the risk of salmonella poisoning will increase).

18. Cats, dogs and even birds can all carry infections which may be dangerous to you so don't let them clamber over surfaces where you prepare or serve food. And if you handle an animal make sure that you wash your hands thoroughly before preparing or eating food. Make sure that you keep feeding dishes and serving utensils intended for animals well away from those which you use. Wash up dishes used by animals in different water.

19. Don't put warm food into the refrigerator — if you do then the temperature inside the fridge may rise to an unsafe level and other food stored there may be spoilt.

20. Make sure that you know how to use all the equipment in your kitchen — and check that your oven, fridge and microwave (if you use one) are all working properly. Be careful to make sure that you follow the manufacturer's instructions carefully

CHAPTER SIX

DRUGS AND HORMONES

In order to maximise their profits modern farmers often use drugs and hormones to keep their animals 'healthy'. The drugs help to reduce the financial loss of animals dying. Since animals are often kept in overcrowded conditions the need for artificial help is often considerable. In addition drugs are frequently used to improve the weight and appearance of animals intended for sale as meat.

Modern, intensive farming techniques mean that animals are usually kept in very cramped and uncomfortable conditions. To keep animals calm tranquillisers are used. And to reduce the risk of infection antibiotics are used. A few years ago antibiotics were used simply to treat sick animals and to prevent illness spreading. There can, of course, be no argument against this. It would be obviously wrong not to treat animals who were ill. But these days antibiotics are quite commonly used in a very different — and indefensible way. In order to prevent infections developing and to encourage a faster than average growth rate antibiotics are routinely added to animal feeds. Nearly half of all the antibiotics currently being manufactured go into animal feeds. Young animals are taken from their mothers at such an early age that they have no chance to acquire any natural immunity by drinking their mother's milk and so they are much more susceptible to disease. It is not at all uncommon for young animals to be kept on antibiotics for the whole of their lives.

There are several dangers with this over-use of antibiotics. First, drug resistant bacteria are already developing. The overuse of antibiotics in farming means that when doctors try to use those drugs to treat sick human patients the drugs simply don't work — the bacteria have become so accustomed to the antibiotics that they are not killed by them. The number of drugs available to doctors has, in this way, been dramatically reduced in recent years. This problem is exacerbated by the fact that when humans eat the meat from animals fed on antibiotics they swallow both the remnants of the antibiotics and the bacteria which have acquired antibiotic resistance. By giving their animals antibiotics modern farmers are endangering the health and indeed the lives of their customers.

People who eat meat are also at risk from the hormones which are commonly used by farmers. Growth hormones are popular because if you give an animal a growth hormone it will grow faster and achieve a heavier weight sooner. In some parts of the world meat which has been prepared with the aid of hormones has officially been banned. However, these bans usually prove to be more technical than realistic and the profits to be made by using hormones to increase the speed at which animals grow means that farmers are secretly often still giving hormones to their animals. The people who eat meat from animals which have been reared with the aid of hormones eventually end up consuming those hormones too. No one knows what effect the hormone residues will have on human consumers of meat.

One of the hormones traditionally used by farmers is diethylstilboestrol. This hormone is popular because it helps to increase the rate at which both sheep and cattle develop. But diethylstilboestrol is a potentially dangerous substance. Shortly after the Second World War it was given to pregnant women who seemed likely to have miscarriages. In the 1970s it was then revealed that the daughters of women who had been given the hormone were prone to develop cancer of the vagina. This was the first time in history that a link had been established between a drug given to one generation and a disease developing in the next generation. Officially farmers are not supposed to use diethylstilboestrol. But farmers do a lot of things which they are not officially supposed to do and just as drug use among athletes is commonplace, so the use of this hormone on farms around the world is common. Doctors have reported that babies and young girls have started to develop breasts — and even started to produce milk of their own — after being fed on milk that has come from cows which have been given hormones. In Italy women noticed that their babies had started developing breasts: this bizarre occurrence was blamed on the use of hormones in meat, after it was found that the women had given their babies baby food manufactured from animals which had been boosted with diethylstilboestrol.

In America the use of hormones is so common that 80% of the cattle reared have been artificially enhanced with the aid of hormones. A single, very cheap hormone pellet can help make an animal put on an extra 22kg of lean meat — while consuming less food than an animal which has not been given a hormone pellet.

The Americans claim that giving hormones to cattle is perfectly safe but beef from such cattle is banned in the EU.

Farmers give six sex hormones to their cattle for exactly the same reason that body-builders and weight-lifters take hormones: to speedily build more muscle. The benefit to a farmer is financial: there is obviously more saleable beef on a heavily muscled cow.

The row, which has been going on for well over a decade, is about whether or not beef taken from cows which have been given extra hormones is safe to eat. Although there is no evidence to show that hormone-soaked beef is safe American farmers say that it is. And that, of course, is good enough for their government. (All governments are as frightened of farmers as they are of any other big commercial group.)

However, European farmers are not allowed to give extra hormones to cattle. And so, not surprisingly, they have put pressure on European politicians to ban the American beef (which, because of the help from the hormones, is cheaper to produce).

The American claim that it is safe to give hormones to cattle is based upon the fact that there is, as yet, not very much scientific proof that it is dangerous to do this.

This is exactly the same spurious argument that is used to defend genetic engineering, microwave ovens and other possible hazards to human health.

Everyone conveniently ignores the fact that it is extremely difficult to prove that something is dangerous when no research has been done to find the truth.

What we do know, however, is that the amount of hormone in 500 grams of meat can be more than a pubertal boy produces in a day. And that's a lot. And sex hormones can and do have a dramatic effect on any human body (and mind).

Moreover, research has been done showing that there is a convincing epidemiological link between one of the six hormones used by American farmers and endometrial and breast cancers. The hormone causes cancer by interfering with a cell's DNA — a process known as genotoxicity. It is generally accepted that there are no safe levels for genotoxic substances.

You might think that would be enough to embarrass the American politicians into telling their farmers to stop using hormones. After all, the incidence of cancer is rising dramatically in the US — and has been doing so for some years.

However, the American farmers (and their government) have taken comfort from the fact that although a joint committee set up by the World Health Organization and the Food and Agriculture Organisation has agreed that one of the hormones in use (estradiol-17-beta) has what it calls 'genotoxic properties', and does cause cancer, it has argued that it is safe to allow people to consume modest amounts of this cancer inducing hormone. Moreover, much to the delight of the Americans, the committee claims to know what the safe level is. You will not be surprised to hear that the American farmers and their government claim that their beef contains less than this safe amount of this known cancer inducing substance.

In my view anyone who eats American beef is playing a modern version of Russian roulette and is exhibiting an extraordinary amount of trust in a group of people (American politicians and American farmers) who have consistently shown that they do not give a fig for human health or human life.

The use of hormones in Europe is illegal but I know of fifteen illegal growth hormones available on the black market in European countries. It seems reasonable to assume that some farmers probably know of the existence of these illegal growth hormones too.

Tranquillisers, hormones and antibiotics are not the only chemicals or drugs which are given to animals — and which are likely to find their way into the bodies of those who eat meat. Farmers use a variety of other chemicals in order to maximise their profits. One chemical is given to animals to kill fly eggs in their manure. The aim is to reduce the number of flies in overcrowded animal sheds but I don't think anyone knows how dangerous this chemical could be to the human consumers of meat taken from these animals. A substance called a prostaglandin is sometimes injected into animals in order to bring them into 'season' at a convenient time.

To all this we must add the fact that animals do produce their own natural hormones — and modern farming techniques often mean that the existence of these hormones may be particularly high. For example, when they are frightened animals produce the hormone adrenalin. Since slaughterhouses are pretty terrifying places there can be little doubt that just before they die animals usually have a lot of adrenalin circulating in their bodies. Just what effect does all that adrenalin have on humans? Your guess is as good as anyone else's.

CHAPTER SEVEN

MAD COW DISEASE

Britain's mad cow disease scandal was caused when farmers turned herbivores into cannibals. It was a direct result of greed. But politicians consistently defended and protected farmers, and for years deliberately hid the truth about this exceptional — but very real — hazard.

When, in 1990, I first warned that mad cow disease could prove to be a major problem (and cause serious health problems — and death — in human beings) I was vilified by the government for 'scaremongering'. When in 1993 I repeated my warning that people who ate beef, and beef products, were taking a real risk with their health Sir Kenneth Calman, at the time Britain's chief medical officer, assured people that beef could safely be eaten by everyone. 'To say that Dr Coleman's views are alarmist would be an understatement,' Calman announced. (Since this senior government spokesman used the word 'alarmist' I feel justified in pointing out that it was politicians who warned us that we were all going to die of AIDS — deliberately creating the biggest false scare of the 20th century.)

When I exclusively revealed that mad cow disease was being transmitted back to sheep by feeding the carcases of cows suffering from mad cow disease to sheep I was again dismissed as a scaremonger. Subsequently, I was once again proved right.

It seems to me that the whole mad cow saga confirms my thesis that far too much decision making in our world is done in the interests of institutions and corporations — and business in general — rather than in the interests of individuals.

Details of how politicians allow farmers to feed their animals are coming to light with greater frequency in the wake of the appalling mad cow disease scandal in the UK.

For example, among the cheap 'foods' fed to cattle and pigs on farms in the US are: human sewage sludge, dead cats and dogs, chicken manure, slaughterhouse waste (blood, bones, intestines), cement kiln dust, old newspapers, waste cardboard, agricultural waste (corn cobs, fruit and vegetable peelings) and old fat from restaurants and grease traps. Those who eat meat are, of course, consuming the residues of all these delectables. What a tribute all this is to the glory of our allegedly sophisticated world.

If it is true (as I believe it is) that we are what we eat then this news should alarm all meat eaters. What farmers choose to include in animal feed is crucial to human health.

ANIMAL FEED

Approximately seven million Americans suffer from food-borne illnesses every year. (The figures for other Western nations are proportionately similar.)

One reason for what is now undeniably a major epidemic is the fact that animal manure remains attached to or mixed with meat which is sent to the shops for human consumption.

Another reason for the food-borne epidemic is the fact that many cooks do not prepare meat properly — often by not cooking it thoroughly.

But the use of animal excrement as animal feed must be another major cause of illness.

The millions of farm animals reared to satisfy the Western world's apparently insatiable demand for meat between them produce an enormous amount of waste. Farm animals in the United

States produce ten times as much waste as the human population and an expert working at the University of Georgia recently pointed out that just seven chickens produce as much manure as one human being. In America, where around seven billion chickens are raised and killed every year, the annual production of excrement now totals in excess of 1.5 billion tons.

Getting rid of this enormous quantity of excrement obviously poses something of a problem to farmers. You simply can't spread it all on the fields as fertiliser. (Getting rid of just some of that excrement by dumping it onto the land is one reason why drinking water supplies are so polluted.)

And so, in an attempt to get rid of all this toxic waste, farmers now frequently mix animal waste into livestock feed. Chicken litter is particularly commonly dealt with in this way (perhaps because its composition makes it easier to deal with — and the quantity of it makes its disposal a real problem).

In some areas of America roughly one in every five chicken farmers now use their chicken manure for cattle feed. Such laws as there are only seem to apply to commercial feed manufacturers and so farmers who keep both chicken and cattle seem to be able to feed chicken manure to cows with impunity. I have no doubt that this same practice is followed in other areas of the world where farmers keep chicken and cattle.

I am convinced that the mixing of chicken manure in with animal feed is an important cause of infection. Chicken commonly carry the salmonella bug (among others). And so the cattle who eat the chicken manure also then become infected with the salmonella.

It is hardly surprising that food borne disease is now commonplace. Food from the US is, of course, imported freely into Britain and other parts of Europe.

MEAT PRODUCTS

Modern regulations allow farmers, meat processors, packers and food companies selling meat to mislead their consumers in a way that would startle people in other industries.

The word 'meat' can include the head, feet, rectum (full or empty), spinal cord and tail of an animal. The term 'meat product' can include the eyeballs and the nose. A package which is labelled as containing pure beef may include fat, rind, gristle and skin. It is commonplace for sausages to include ground up tonsils, fat, bone, cartilage and intestines (with or without the contents). The people selling meat and meat products use flavourings and colourings to disguise what they are selling. Faecal matter is an advantage — it adds extra weight. Water and polyphosphates are injected into the animal's dead body at high pressure in order to increase the weight of the animal (and the profit to the farmer).

MORE MEAT WORRIES

The enormous demand for meat these days means that every day huge numbers of animals are killed and 'processed'. In theory the killing should be clean, fast, painless and hygienic. It is none of those things. The killing invariably goes on in huge sheds where cross infection is commonplace and where there is little or no time to clear away blood or faecal matter. Chickens are routinely killed in batches of thousands at a time. Inevitably carcasses become infected. Cross infection in slaughterhouses is common. Contamination with faecal matter is commonplace and animals which are ill, infected or cancerous are killed and 'processed' into the food chain for humans. People who eat meat could easily end up eating a lump of cancer.

Before animals are killed they are usually made unconscious. This is done either with a special type of pistol which fires a captive steel bolt or by passing an electric current through the animal's brain.

Then, when they are supposedly unconscious, the animals are killed by having their throats slit. (The men who work in the slaughterhouses call this 'sticking', 'bleeding out', or — if they are feeling unusually literate — 'exsanguination'.)

However, the animals aren't always unconscious when their throats are cut. Approximately 6% of cattle are not properly stunned before their throats are cut. And many animals wake up in time to see what is happening to them. Worst of all, however, are the practices in slaughterhouses which cater to Jews and Muslims. Here, for some (to me quite incomprehensible) reason, animals are fully conscious when their throats are cut. In Britain alone approximately 50,000 to 60,000 cattle and calves, 25,000 to 30,000 sheep and lambs and millions of chickens, turkey and hens are alive when their throats are cut so that Jews can eat kosher meat. Cattle can take up to six minutes to die this way.

Approximately 4,000 animals die every minute of every working day in slaughterhouses in the United Kingdom.

CHAPTER EIGHT

FOOD IRRADIATION — FACTS YOU SHOULD KNOW

Food is often expensive and time consuming to grow. It is, however, often more expensive to transport, package and store. So to avoid the inevitable wastage (and financial cost) of food 'spoiling', manufacturers and distributors use a wide variety of techniques to preserve and to extend the shelf life of the food they sell.

Drying, smoking and salting are among the oldest and best-established techniques but these methods do not always work and are not always entirely safe. Not long ago a report from the Food and Agriculture Organization and the World Health Organization concluded that 'illness due to contaminated food is perhaps the most widespread health problem in the contemporary world'.

There is no doubt that the incidence of food borne disease has gone up dramatically during the last few years. Much to the consternation of the food manufacturers — and their scientists — many of the chemicals previously used to preserve food are now under suspicion of damaging human health.

Because of the problems associated with chemicals used to preserve food a new technique — irradiation — is now being used to preserve food.

The technique used is very simple.

The food to be preserved is radiated — exposed to the same sort of radiation that is more normally used to take X-rays of broken bones and to treat some types of cancer. One of the substances used to irradiate food is extracted from waste products obtained from nuclear plants. The X-rays kill fungi, bacteria and insects that might otherwise make food spoil.

This technique is proving to be very popular with food companies. They do not, of course, like it when food goes rotten and has to be thrown away. 'Spoilt' food costs the industry huge sums of money every year.

But the 64,000 dollar question is: Is radiation safe?

Those who advocate radiation claim that it is safer than using chemical preservatives.

But the truth is that we won't know whether irradiated food is safe to eat until a large number of human beings have eaten it for a long time.

Here are just some of the possible problems which could be associated with irradiated food.

1. Irradiation can reduce the number of vitamins in food. How much will this affect the people who eat irradiated food? I don't think anyone knows yet. We will probably have to wait another twenty years to find out.

2. Irradiation does not kill all the bugs in food. After treatment any bugs which have survived in the food may simply start to multiply again. For example, irradiating food doesn't necessarily protect the consumer against botulism, a frequently fatal and particularly nasty form of food-borne disease.

3. Exposing food to ionizing radiation can result in the production of special chemical compounds called radiolytic products. These compounds will, of course, be eaten. But will they be safe to eat? I don't think anyone knows the answer to that question yet. We will probably have to wait another twenty years to find out.

4. Irradiated food may taste and smell differently to ordinary food. Apart from the obvious disadvantage associated with this there is another hazard: will consumers be able to recognise when food is bad if it smells and tastes different anyway? At present the smell and taste of food is often a useful guide to its edibility. I don't think anyone knows the answer to those questions yet.

5. The individuals who work in the food irradiating plants may be exposed to danger — in just the same way that the first radiologists were exposed to danger because the hazards associated with the technique being used were not fully understood. How dangerous will food irradiation be to people working in the food industry? I don't think anyone knows the answer to that question yet. We will probably have to wait another twenty years to find out.

6. Many of the foods that seem to be most suitable for irradiation — and this includes such staples as fruit and vegetables — are the foods which are normally the healthiest and which provide many people with vital nutrients. These foods are particularly suitable for irradiation because they go off quite quickly if they are not 'preserved'. But how many essential nutrients will be damaged by irradiation? And will consumers be turned away from these excellent foods if they know that they have been irradiated? I don't think anyone knows the answer to that question yet. We will probably have to wait another twenty years to find out.

7. Even if one country brings in laws to control irradiation — and to ensure that consumers are told when the food they are buying has been irradiated — it will probably be difficult to stop importers moving foods around the world after they have been given large

doses of radiation. How will the consumer know how much radiation a food has been given? How much is too much? I don't think anyone knows the answer to those questions yet. We will probably have to wait another twenty years to find out.

8. Irradiated foods may look fresh even though they are not. The result may be that you will buy food that is past its best. You will, therefore, suffer twice: you will be eating 'bad' food and you will be eating food that has been irradiated.

I am convinced that food irradiation is neither necessary nor welcome. There are, in my view, far too many opportunities for abuse and far too many potential pitfalls.

My advice is to avoid any food that has been irradiated. Try to do most of your shopping at shops which you know do not sell irradiated food. And try to eat out in restaurants which do not serve irradiated food.

CHAPTER NINE

MICROWAVE OVENS

It isn't just the poor quality of the food we buy which makes us ill — damaging our immune systems and making us vulnerable to infections and to cancer.

The way we prepare our food can also have a dramatic effect on our health. Overcooking food can destroy the vitamin content, for example.

And consider the microwave oven.

There are millions of microwave ovens in use around the world. Unlike traditional ovens they work by using short wave electromagnetic radiation to heat up food.

But, although microwave ovens are widely sold, widely used and sit in millions of kitchens heating (and affecting) the food that people eat, neither governments nor manufacturers seem keen to provide or publish information showing exactly how safe these products are.

In 1998 *The Journal of Natural Science* published an extremely significant paper dealing with the effects of microwaves on humans. The paper, was written by William Kopp, who worked at the Atlantis Rising Educational Center in Portland, Oregon from 1977 to 1979 and who, while working there, gathered together early documents detailing what was then known about the harmful effects of microwave ovens on human beings.

By writing this paper Kopp annoyed a powerful lobby. According to the *Journal of Natural Science* he subsequently changed his name and disappeared. This may sound dramatic but I have met another researcher who examined the dangers of microwave ovens who has been subjected to threats, and whose attempts to publicise the truth about microwave ovens has been met with lawsuits and other attempts to silence him.

Kopp reported that microwave ovens were originally developed by the Nazis for use by mobile support operations during the planned invasion of the Soviet Union. The aim was to eliminate the logistical problem of finding cooking fuels — as well as to cut down cooking times. The initial German research was conducted by the Germans in 1942-3 at the Humboldt-Universitat zu Berlin.

After the end of World War II, wrote Kopp, the Allies discovered the medical research which related to microwave ovens. Experimental microwave equipment was transferred both to the US War Department and to the Soviet Union for investigation. In the Soviet Union research work was done at the Institute of Radio Technology at Kinsk and the Institute of Radio Technology at Rajasthan.

It was in the Soviet Union that most of the research was done and published. And it was the Soviet Union, reported Kopp, which found that a human did not even need to ingest microwaved food substances to be in danger, because even exposure to the energy field itself was sufficient to cause serious adverse side effects.

Kopp pointed out that Soviet scientists were so alarmed about the hazards associated with microwave ovens that the Soviet Union produced a state law in 1976 which forbad the use of any microwave apparatus.

Here is a list of some of the adverse effects listed by the Soviet scientists back in the 1970s as having been observed when human beings were exposed to microwaves:

* A destabilisation in the production of hormones &
maintenance of hormone balance in both males and females.

* Brainwave disturbance in the alpha, theta and delta wave signal
patterns.

* A breakdown of the human 'life energy field'.

* A degeneration and destabilisation of internal cellular membrane
properties.

* A degeneration and breakdown of electrical nerve impulses within
the cerebrum.

* A long term cumulative loss of vital energies within humans,
animals and plants which were located within a 500 m radius of the
operational equipment.

* Long lasting residual effects in the nervous system and lymphatic
systems.

* Negative psychological effects (produced as a result of the brain
wave pattern changes) which included: loss of memory, loss of
ability to concentrate, changes in intellect and emotional responses
and sleep disturbances.

More recently obtained evidence seems to confirm that the danger of microwave ovens is not confined to what happens to the food that is cooked inside them.

Despite the protective shields with which they may be fitted microwave ovens give out extra low frequency electromagnetic fields which may be high enough to produce lymphatic cancer in children.

And when white blood cells are exposed to the sort of electromagnetic fields given out by microwave ovens their ability to fight disease may be reduced dramatically.

Worldwide there are now over 7,000 scientific publications in existence dealing with the health damage caused by short wave transmitters. The damage to cells and cell membranes caused by electromagnetic fields has been well known to scientists for years. (Although, naturally, the electrical and telecommunications industries have steadfastly followed the early example of the tobacco industry and denied that their products could possibly cause cancer or, indeed, any other serious health problem.)

The scientists who examined food which had been cooked in microwave ovens came across a number of serious problems. Here is a summary, listed in William Kopp's paper in the *Journal of Natural Science* of some of the serious changes which have been identified:

* In a statistically high percentage of persons, microwaved foods caused stomach and intestinal cancerous growths, as well as a gradual breakdown of the function of the digestive and excretive systems.

* When meat was heated sufficiently for eating the cancer causing agent d-nitrosodiethanoloamine was created.

* Cancer-causing agents in milk and cereal grains were produced.

* Eating food that had been heated by microwave resulted in a higher percentage of cancer cells within the blood.

* Microwave emissions caused serious alterations to frozen fruits when they were thawed in a microwave oven.

* Changes took place in raw, cooked or frozen vegetables when they were exposed to microwaves for 'extremely short' periods of time.

* Because of chemical changes which had taken place in food that was heated in a microwave oven, human lymphatic systems malfunctioned with a result that the human body did not adequately protect itself against some types of cancerous growth.

In addition, scientists have found that microwave heating also causes 'significant decreases in the nutritive value of all foods researched'.

Among other serious problems they found that there was a drop in the availability of B complex vitamins, vitamin C, vitamin E and essential minerals in foods that had been heated in a microwave oven.

The September 1998 edition of *The Journal of Natural Science* contained yet more evidence drawing attention to the possible hazards associated with microwave ovens:

* In 1990 researchers in Berlin found that all the microwave ovens it tested emitted microwaves while operating.

* As far as microwaves are concerned the most sensitive part of the body is the lens in the eye. Anyone who operates a microwave oven (particularly at eye level) which leaks could go blind.

* Studies with broccoli and carrots have revealed that cell structures are destroyed in the microwave oven. (In conventional ovens the cell walls remain intact.)

* Cooking in a microwave oven creates free radicals — known to be a possible cancer trigger.

* Food cooked in a microwave oven may be cooked unevenly — leaving possible 'cold spots' inside the food. This may result in the possible development of listeria or salmonella infection.

* Water samples were heated, both conventionally and in a microwave oven. The water samples were then used to help grain germinate. Grain did not germinate when in contact with water which had been heated in a microwave oven.

* At the end of the 1980s it was reported that there was an increased incidence of malformations among children of mothers exposed to microwave ovens.

* In 1991 a patient in Oklahoma is alleged to have died of anaphylaxis after receiving a blood transfusion with blood warmed in a microwave oven. It is claimed that the microwave irradiation had altered the blood and thereby caused the patient's death.

* Scientists have discovered that microwaving human breast milk at high temperatures produced a marked decrease in activity of all the tested anti-infective factors naturally present in breast milk. The growth of E.coli was 18 times that observed in normal human breast milk.

* In 1989 the Swiss biologist Dr Hans Hertel, together with another researcher, conducted a study on the effects of microwaved food which proved that food which had been cooked in a microwave oven caused significant changes in the blood. The authors noted that these changes indicated the beginning of a pathological process (e.g. the beginning of cancer). Afterwards the second researcher, who had worked with Dr Hertel, disassociated himself from the results and his earlier interpretation of the results. In a private letter to Dr Hertel the second researcher admitted that he feared 'consequences' and that the safety of his family was more important to him than anything else.

The October/November 1998 issue of *Nexus* magazine reported that a physicist had presented research showing that the human body generates and emits its own low intensity radiation.

The physicist claimed that the human body's metabolism generates its own electromagnetic field. The weak emissions of light which are produced by the body are an outward sign of an orderly, functioning metabolism. This research opens up another series of questions about the effect external sources of microwave radiation may have on living tissues.

It seems perfectly clear to me that microwave ovens should be banned. And any such ban should only be lifted if the manufacturers are prepared to do research which either shows that these original research findings are inaccurate or shows that there are ways to counteract the problems.But a ban on microwave ovens seems about as likely as the medical profession standing up and admitting that the orthodox approach to cancer treatment has failed.

The manufacture and sale of microwave ovens is now big business and these convenient items have become fixtures in canteens, restaurants, hotels and homes all over the world.

In *The Journal of Natural Science* Dr Hertel points out that: '...research of the biological effects of electromagnetic fields on life, especially connected with technical microwaves, is successfully being suppressed. Such research projects are, therefore, only possible on a private basis while the relevant authorities do everything they can to keep the findings from the public, denying them, making them look ridiculous or dismissing them as non scientific.'

I believe that Dr Hertel is absolutely right.

Mainstream newspapers, magazines, television and radio have consistently ignored or denied the threat posed by microwave ovens. Politicians have refused to ask for these devices to be properly tested.

In my experience, attempts to publicise the possible hazards (and the fact that the industry making and selling microwave ovens has never done adequate testing on the effects on human health) seem to have been met with more concern for the health of the microwave industry than for the health and safety of consumers.

Back in January 1990 I warned, in a newspaper article, that thousands could die every year from the effect of food cooked in microwave ovens.

I pointed out that it could be 10, 20 or 30 years before the damage done by microwave ovens could be fully assessed and added that I was appalled that manufacturers had not fully tested microwave ovens.

In the UK the British Broadcasting Corporation (BBC) subsequently broadcast a programme attacking me for this warning and blaming me as the source of a 'scare' about the heating of milk in microwave ovens. My offer to appear on the programme to discuss the issue and defend my point of view was rejected.

(Rather to my surprise, my complaint about the BBC's *Food and Drink* programme was duly upheld by the Broadcasting Complaints Commission which described the BBC programme as 'unfair to Dr Coleman'.)

CHAPTER TEN

GENETICALLY ALTERED FOOD

Science has, during the last few decades, presented us with a steadily increasing and apparently endless variety of moral dilemmas and practical threats. The subject of genetic engineering is a perfect example of how politicians have betrayed us all and are, through their refusal to take on big industry, threatening our very future.

In two decades or so genetic engineering has evolved so rapidly as a branch of science (if science is the right word for a form of alchemy which seems to pay little or no attention to logic or research) that the future of our species is now threatened. Genetic engineering enables scientists to transfer genes between species in an entirely unnatural way. Human genes can be transferred to pigs, sheep, fish or bacteria. And genes from bacteria, slugs, elephants, fish, tomatoes and anything else can be put into human beings.

Genetic engineering started in the 1970s. The technique involves putting genes from one species into another species. In order to do this the genetic engineers put the genes they want to move into viruses. They then put the virus into the animal or plant which is to be the recipient. Genetic engineering is nothing at all like conventional breeding techniques (such as are used by dog breeders who want dogs with very floppy ears or by people who want to grow black tulips).

Listen to the boastful, extraordinarily arrogant claims of genetic scientists and you might believe that they had all the answers to hunger and disease. They talk grandly about eradicating starvation by creating new high yield, pest resistant versions of existing foods and manipulating genes to banish physical ailments, aggression and depression. They will, they say, be able to eradicate homosexuality, control the overpopulation problem, purify water supplies, remove crime from our streets and deal with deforestation. Genetic engineers have even talked of modified strains of bacteria able to eat up plastics, heavy metals and other toxic wastes.

Vast amounts of money (at least $3 billion) have been poured into identifying the human genome (the genetic blue print for human life). There has even been talk that we will be able to clone ourselves so that we need never die.

Moral and ethical questions have been brushed aside as the unnecessary anxieties of ignorant Luddites who either do not understand what is going on or are temperamentally opposed to progress.

But if it all sounds too good to be true — and all rather reminiscent of the sort of cheap promises with which confidence tricksters make their money — that is because it simply isn't true. Genetic scientists don't have the answers to any of our problems. On the contrary they have created a hugely successful money making myth which keeps them in fat grants and huge salaries. (It is important not to underestimate the importance of money in the world of genetic engineering. The world market for biotechnology products is growing at 30% a year.)

None of this would matter too much if what they were doing was as harmless as it is useless. But harmless it is definitely not! Fiddling around with genes is an exceedingly hazardous business. Simply inserting a gene from one creature into another can cause cancer.

Genetic engineering is not something we can simply ignore until the thousands who are making the grand claims areexposed as fraudsters, or until their poorly based pseudoscience falls out of fashion. It is time that the insane burblings of the geneticists were exposed for what they are. I have been writing about the horrors of genetic engineering for over twenty years — since I first realised that scientists were making promises it was clear they couldn't keep — but most doctors, critics and journalists have so far been too frightened (or ignorant) to oppose the torrent of undiluted praise for genetic engineering and point a firm finger at just another invisible suit of clothes for the same old naked Emperor.

When genetic engineering first hit the headlines, the public was promised that there would be strict rules about just what could and could not be done. But the rules that were intended to protect us have been bent, pushed aside and ignored. Regulations were, it was claimed, slowing down progress, interfering with the competitiveness of the developing new industry and getting in the way of individual scientists keen to get on with their plan for improving the world. It is wrong, say the scientists, to try to ban new thinking or new research.

Genetic engineers claim that there is no need for caution and that only the narrow minded and the reactionary have reservations about this exciting new branch of scientific endeavour.

But the fact is that the genetic engineering industry has even succeeded in 'persuading' politicians and administrators that there is no need to segregate genetically engineered produce from naturally grown produce.

The risks associated with genetic engineering are numerous and widespread. There is little doubt that genetic engineering is at least partly responsible for the problem of antibiotic-resistant organisms. And there is even less doubt that genetic engineering is responsible for some, and possibly many, of the new infective organisms now threatening human health.

Under normal circumstances viruses are species specific. A virus that attacks a cat will not attack a human being. And a virus that attacks a human being will not attack a cow. But the genetic engineers have changed all that. They have deliberately glued together different bits of viruses in order to cross species barriers. These genetically engineered viruses can then become virulent again. Genetically engineered viruses are extremely infectious. None of this happens by accident — this is how genetic engineering works.

Naturally, the men and women in white coats who were convinced that they knew best ('Trust us — nothing can go wrong') have been releasing genetic material that they have been fiddling with into the environment for years. A year or two ago we thought that the dumping of waste chemicals was bad news. But the dumping of genetic misshapes and off-cuts will, I believe, create a problem infinitely larger than the dumping of chemical waste or even nuclear waste. Genes, once they start moving and reproducing, can keep spreading, recombining and affecting new species for ever. Once the door has been opened it cannot be shut. And the door has been opened.

'Don't worry!' said the genetic engineers, when this problem was identified. 'Genetic material is easily digested by gut enzymes.'

Sadly, they were wrong about that too.

Genetic material can survive a journey through an intestine and find its way, via the blood stream, into all sorts of body cells. And once inside a new body the genetic material can begin to affect host cells. If you eat a genetically engineered tomato the foreign genes in the tomato could end up in your cells. Cancer is an obvious possible consequence of this. Exactly what are the risks? I'm afraid that your guess is as good as mine. And our guesses are just as good as the guesses made by genetic engineers. They don't have the foggiest idea what will happen. But they know that something terrible could happen.

Readers will, I am sure, have realised that this poses a new and startling question: what about the altered genetic material in new types of food? What happens to genetically altered food when it is eaten? Will the altered genes find their way into our own genetic material? Could genetically engineered food cause cancer? Could genetically engineered food affect the human immune system?

Asking the questions is easy. But no one knows the answers.

Genetically engineered foods have already been shown to produce allergy problems — and to be toxic. One major hazard is that plants which have been genetically engineered to be resistant to disease may be more likely to produce allergy problems. A soya bean genetically engineered with a gene from a brazil nut was found to cause allergy problems when eaten by people sensitive to Brazil nuts. A strain of yeast, genetically altered in order to ferment more quickly, acquired cancer inducing qualities. Contaminants in an amino acid produced by a Japanese company led to 1,500 people falling ill and to the deaths of 37 individuals.

And yet politicians have done nothing to protect the public. The manufacturers of genetically engineered foods do not have to identify foods that have been genetically engineered. No one tests genetically engineered foods to see whether or not they are particularly likely to cause allergy problems. The new food is tested when it is put onto the market. You and I are the unwitting test subjects. Even drug companies have to do some tests before they can launch new products. Food companies seem to be entirely free of controls.

Amazingly, the politicians and administrators whom we pay to protect us allow the manufacturers to get away with the argument that it would be impossible to separate and identify genetically engineered foods. 'Segregation of bulk commodities is not scientifically justified and is economically unrealistic,' said the industries involved in genetic engineering. 'Certainly!' said the politicians and the bureaucrats. 'If you say so.' The US government announced that it would not tolerate the segregation or labelling of genetically engineered crops. The US government has stated: 'We do not find any scientific evidence to support the assertion that bio-engineered foods are inherently less safe. Therefore they should not be singled out for special labelling requirements.' In my view this must rank as one of the most hollow and absurd statements of the century since as far as I am aware no one has done any clinical investigations to find out whether or not bio-engineered foods are safe, a bit unsafe or completely deadly.

European politicians do not have the guts to stand up to American politicians. They are frightened that if they upset the Americans the Americans will introduce trade embargoes. (The American government, desperate as ever not to annoy big American companies, warned food companies that if they label their products as not containing genetically engineered food they will not be looked upon favourably if they attempt to market their products in the US.)

The problems are only just beginning but already they are frightening. Potatoes and oilseed rape were genetically engineered to be resistant to herbicide. The resistance spread to weeds within a single growing season. Thanks to the irresponsible overuse and abuse of pesticides, and the widespread introduction of crops genetically engineered to produce 'natural' insecticides, more than 1,000 agricultural pests have now acquired so much resistance that they are immune to chemical control. Crops which have been genetically engineered to tolerate herbicides have already begun to make weeds immune to the same herbicides.

If the big seed companies and the politicians have their way then within a year or two farmers throughout the world will be growing the same variety of genetically engineered soya, the same type of genetically engineer potato and the same genetically engineered corn. That is not a prediction which is difficult to make. It is exactly what the big seed manufacturers are planning. And when the world's single crop of soya/potatoes/corn is destroyed by an insect or plant disease which is immune to every pesticide known to man (and remember there are already 1,000 insects and plant diseases which satisfy that requirement) countless millions around the world will die of starvation.

I strongly suggest that you refuse to buy — or eat — food that has had its genetic composition changed in any way.

CHAPTER ELEVEN

FOODS THAT CAUSE CANCER

An A to Z of Evidence

You may be surprised to hear that there is now clear medical and scientific evidence available to show that nothing, not even tobacco, influences your chances of developing cancer as much as the food you choose to eat. It is estimated that between 30% and 60% of all cancers are caused by what you choose to eat. Doctors, scientists and supporters of the cancer industry claim that the battle against cancer will only be won with the aid of more money. They claim that in order to obtain the information we need we must spend, spend, spend. But that isn't true. It is not more knowledge we need (we have, as I pointed out in *Paper Doctors* nearly twenty years ago, already amassed far more knowledge than we will ever use in our lifetime), but the ability and courage and determination to use the knowledge we already have.

Back in 1982 the National Research Council in the United States of America published a technical report entitled Diet, Nutrition and Cancer which showed that diet was probably the single most important factor in the development of cancer, and that there was evidence linking cancers of the breast, colon and prostate to particular foods or types of food.

It is a scandal of astonishing proportions that a majority of the population still do not know about these vitally important and well established links. It is an even bigger scandal that a majority of the medical profession are unaware of these links too. Most doctors I have spoken to — even recently qualified ones — still dismiss the idea of a food/cancer link as mumbo- jumbo nonsense, preferring to rely entirely on prescription drugs, radiotherapy and surgery as 'treatments' for cancer. The average medical student probably spends more time staring down a microscope at histology slides than he or she spends studying the importance and significance of nutrition.

After he had seen an earlier edition of this book, one doctor sent me a very indignant letter, asking me whether I thought it was ethical to publish such statements as 'Between a third and a half of all cancers are caused by eating the wrong types of food' and 'You can dramatically reduce your chances of developing cancer of the breast, cancer of the prostate, cancer of the colon, cancer of the ovary or cancer of the uterus.'

(After I had sent him details of a small amount of the evidence upon which I had based those statements, the doctor wrote back and apologised.)

I checked one large (over 1,000 pages) recently published medical textbook and found that the chapter on cancer summed up the role of food as a causal agent in just one, rather short sentence. I find this all extremely difficult to understand. I have been studying scientific research papers for over two decades and I have never seen such convincing research as that which shows the links between particular types of food and particular types of cancer.

It is not uncommon for new drugs to be launched after clinical trials which may have involved relatively small numbers of patients. In my book *Betrayal of Trust* I pointed out that the number of patients studied in clinical trials before a drug is marketed is, on average, only 1,480 — and that the final, total,overall figure is sometimes much less than this.

In contrast some of the individual research projects which have been published showing links between food and cancer have involved tens of thousands of patients.

I have absolutely no doubt that if these undeniable links had been publicised by the responsible authorities (in medicine as elsewhere the phrase 'responsible authorities' is, I fear, oxymoronic) countless millions of lives and an enormous amount of agony and distress could — and would — have been avoided.

The suppression of this information by a greedy and conscience-free food industry, compliant revenue conscious politicians, a cancer industry dominated by grant hungry researchers and an uncaring, drug company dominated medical profession has, I sincerely believe, led to more deaths than any war in history.

Since the early 1980s the amount of evidence linking diet to cancer has grown steadily. In 1990 even the British Medical Association, hardly an organisation which would be widely described as revolutionary, supported the view that there is a link between food and cancer. Their published view was that 35% of cancers, just over a third, were caused by the natural constituents of food and that another 1% of cancers were caused by food additives.

Other organisations suggest that the link between food and cancer is even higher. The National Academy of Sciences in the United States, founded in 1863 by Act of Congress to serve as an official adviser to the US government in all matters of science and technology, has reported that researchers have estimated that almost 60% of women's cancers and a little more than 40% of men's cancers are related to nutritional factors.

Because I recognise that many readers may be sceptical about the claim that there is a strong link between diet and food (such scepticism will undoubtedly be enhanced by the fact that neither

111

governments nor the medical profession have made much, if any, effort to publicise these links) I have in this chapter summarised just some of the scientific evidence which supports this claim.

My previous efforts to publicise the health values of eating a low fat, meatless diet have been consistently confronted by scepticism and opposition. It is my hope that this summary of just some of the most important available evidence supporting the contention that certain foods are a risk factor in the development of cancer will help settle this particular controversy permanently and may, perhaps, help other writers who may be tempted to tell their readers the truth about food and cancer.

I must emphasise that this list is not intended to be comprehensive. I have accumulated a list of several hundred scientific papers and journal articles dealing with the links between food and cancer (and many thousands more dealing with food and other disorders) and this list is merely intended to be representative — and to provide you with some idea of the breadth and importance of the available evidence.

If you would like to study even more evidence linking food to cancer (and many other diseases) then I heartily recommend the book *Nutritional Influences on Illness: A sourcebook of clinical research*, written by Melvyn R. Werbach MD and published by Thorsons. In a remarkably comprehensive and quite fascinating book Dr Werbach has listed and summarised thousands of clinical studies and scientific reports. He reports that: 'The cancers most closely associated with nutritional factors are breast and endometrial cancer in women, prostate cancer in men and gastrointestinal cancer', points out that 'the value of a low fat, high fibre diet in cancer prevention is well documented' and notes that 'avoidance of smoked, pickled and salt cured foods' has been shown...to be beneficial in preventing cancers of the gastrointestinal tract.'

Dr Werbach adds that 'there is early evidence that certain precancerous changes may be reversible with supplementation'. He reports that cervical dysplasia may possibly be reversed with folic acid supplements, that calcium supplements may help 'reduce the number of rapidly proliferating cells in the colonic epithelium in patients with family histories of colon cancer and elevated numbers of such cells compared to controls' and that Vitamin A or beta-carotene reduce the percent of genetically damaged cells inside the cheek when betel quid, a tobacco-like plant mixture is chewed regularly.'

Exhibit A

Title

Calorie-Providing Nutrients and Risk of Breast Cancer

Authors

Paolo Toniolo (Epidemiology Unit, Istituto Nazionale per lo Studio e la Cura dei Tumori, Milan, Italy and Department of Environmental Medicine, New York University Medical Center, New York, USA), Elio Riboli (Unit of Analytical Epidemiology, International Agency for Research on Cancer, Lyon, France), Fulvia Protta (Pathology Service, Ospedale Maggiore S. Giovanni, Turin, Italy), Martine Charrel (Unit of Analytical Epidemiology, International Agency for Research on Cancer, Lyon, France), Alberto M Cappa (Pathology Service, Ospedale Maggiore S. Giovanni, Turin, Italy)

Source

Journal of the National Cancer Institute

Date

February 15th 1989

Report

This study, which was conducted in the province of Vercelli in northwestern Italy where there is a moderately high incidence of breast cancer, was designed to investigate the role of diet in breast cancer and 'to test the primary hypothesis that fat and proteins from animal sources are associated with increased risk of breast cancer.'

The researchers questioned 250 women with breast cancer and a random sample of 499 women from the general population, using a structured questionnaire to identify the types and quantities of food each woman consumed.

After reporting that they had 'found evidence that the intake of total fat, saturated fat or proteins of animal origin is positively associated with the risk of breast cancer in women' the researchers reported that their 'findings had suggested that during adult life a reduction in total fat to less than 30% of calorie intake, of saturated fat to less than 10% of calorie intake and of animal proteins to less than 6% may lead to a substantial reduction in the incidence of breast cancer in population subgroups with high intake of saturated fat and animal proteins in agreement with some dietary recommendations that have been made.'

'These data,' said the researchers, 'suggest that during adult life a reduction in dietary intake of fat and proteins of animal origin may contribute to a substantial reduction in the incidence of breast cancer in population subgroups with high intake of animal products.'

Exhibit B

Title

Dietary Habits and Prognostic Factors in Breast Cancer

Authors

Lars-Erik Holm (Department of Cancer Prevention, Karolinska Hospital, Stockholm, Sweden), Eva Callmer (Department of Medical Nutrition, Huddinge Hospital, Huddinge, Sweden), Marie-Louise Hjalmar (Department of General Oncology, Danderyd Hospital, Danderyd, Sweden), Elizabet Lidbrink (Department of General Oncology, South Hospital, Stockholm, Sweden), Bo Nilsson (Department of Cancer Epidemiology, Karolinska Hospital, Stockholm, Sweden, Lambert Skoog (Department of Clinical Cytology, Karolinska Hospital, Stockholm, Sweden).

Source

Journal of the National Cancer Institute

Date

August 16th 1989

Report

The link between dietary fat and breast tumours was first described in 1942. Since then many other scientists have published papers detailing this link in further detail. 'Dietary fat has been suggested as an etiological factor in human breast cancer because of the high correlation between national per capita fat consumption and breast cancer incidence,' begin the authors of this paper whose study included 240 women who had surgery for breast cancer between the years of 1983 and 1986 in Stockholm, Sweden. All the women involved in this study were aged between 50 and 65 at the time that their cancers were diagnosed. After analysing their results the authors of this paper concluded: 'The results of this study of mainly postmenopausal women and some premenopausal women suggest that dietary habits have an impact on the prognosis of breast cancer.'

'Study results indicate that dietary factors may act in breast carcinogenesis,' continued the authors in their discussion of their results. 'Several studies have found that these factors also operate after diagnosis of the tumour, suggesting that dietary habits are important even after a successful primary treatment. The results of this study suggest that dietary patterns of the Western world (e.g. high fat intake and low consumption of carbohydrates and fiber) affect certain prognostic factors in breast cancer, such as tumour size and oestrogen receptor content of the tumour.'

Exhibit C

Title

A Case-Control Study of Prostatic Cancer With Reference to Dietary Habits

Authors

Kenji Oishi, Kenichiro Okada, Osamu Yoshida, Hirohiko Yamabe, Yoshiyuki Ohno, Richard B Hayes and Fritz H. Schroeder; (these authors were from the Department of Urology, Kyoto University, Kyoto, Japan; Laboratory of Anatomic Pathology, Kyoto University Hospital, Japan; Department of Public Health, Medical School, Nagoya City University, Nagoya, Japan; Department of Urology, Faculty of Medicine, Erasmus University Rotterdam, The Netherlands.)

Source

The Prostate

Date

1988

Report

In 1950 the incidence of prostatic cancer in Japan was about 0.4 per 100,000 male members of the population but by 1963 it had increased to 2.0 per 100,000 and by 1975 it was 2.5 per 100,000.

Observers have suggested that this increase (which is not unique, for increases in the incidence of cancer of the lung, cancer of the

116

breast and cancer of the colon have also occurred in recent years) may be linked to the Westernisation of Japanese eating habits. During recent years the consumption of fat, animal protein, eggs, dairy products and oil have all increased considerably in Japan.

This study was of sufferers from prostatic cancer from 1981 to 1984 and patients suffering from benign prostatic hypertrophy (non cancerous prostate enlargement) and was conducted to find the risk factors for prostatic cancer. 'Two well trained nutritionists and one urologist interviewed each subject at the time of hospital admission'.

The findings included: 'Low daily intake of beta-carotene ... were significantly correlated with prostatic cancer development.'

Exhibit D

Title

Relation of Meat, Fat and Fiber Intake To The Risk of Colon Cancer in a Prospective Study Among Women

Authors

Walter C. Willett M.D, Meir J. Stampfer M.D., Graham A. Colditz M.D., Bernard A. Rosner Ph.D., and Frank E. Speizer M.D. from the Channing Laboratory, Department of Medicine, Harvard Medical School and Brigham and Women's Hospital, the Department of Preventive Medicine, Harvard Medical School and the Departments of Epidemiology, Nutrition and Biostatistics at the Harvard School of Public Health, all in Boston in the United States of America.

Source

The New England Journal of Medicine

Date

December 13th 1990

Report

The authors of this paper began by pointing out that in Western countries cancer rates are up to ten times as high as they are in many Far Eastern and developing countries. For many years doctors and scientists have noted rapid increases in rates of colon cancer among men and women migrating from low risk areas to high risk areas and these observations have suggested that the large differences which exist may be due to environmental causes rather than genetic causes.

The authors pointed out that two general dietary hypotheses have evolved in recent decades: firstly, that dietary fat, particularly from animal sources, increases the risk of colon cancer and secondly, that the intake of fibre reduces the risk.

This study involved observing 88,751 women between the ages of 34 and 59 for six years. The women, none of whom had any history of cancer, inflammatory bowel disease or familial polyposis, completed a questionnaire about their eating habits in 1980. By the year 1986 a total of 150 cases of coloncancer had been noted.

The researchers concluded that 'animal fat was positively associated with the risk of colon cancer' but that 'no association was found for vegetable fat'. The researchers found that women who ate beef, pork or lamb as a main dish every day were more likely to develop cancer of the colon than were women who ate beef, pork or lamb as a main dish less than once a month. It was also found that processed meats and liver were also 'significantly associated with increased risk'.

The ratio of the intake of red meat to the intake of chicken and fish was particularly strongly associated with an increased incidence of colon cancer,' concluded the researchers, who also noted that 'a low intake of fiber from fruits appeared to contribute to the risk of colon cancer, but this relation was not statistically independent of meat intake.'

'These prospective data provide evidence for the hypothesis that a high intake of animal fat increases the risk of colon cancer,' said the researchers, 'and they support existing recommendations to substitute fish and chicken for meats high in fat.'

Exhibit E

Title

Dietary Fat Consumption and Survival Among Women With Breast Cancer

Authors

David I. Gregorio, Department of Social and Preventive Medicine, State University of New York, Buffalo, New York, United States of America; Lawrence J. Emrich, Department of Biomathematics, Roswell Park Memorial Institute, Buffalo, New York, United States of America; Saxon Graham, Department of Social and Preventive Medicine, State University of New York, Buffalo, New York, United States of America; James R. Marshall, Department of Social and Preventive Medicine, State University of New York, Buffalo, New York, United States of America, and Takuma Nemoto, Department of Breast Surgery, RoswellPark Memorial Institute, Buffalo, New York, United States of America

Source

Journal of the National Cancer Institute

Date

July 1985

Report

The researchers estimated monthly fat consumption for a total of 854 patients who completed dietary intake interviews when they were admitted to hospital and subsequently estimated that 24% of the women consumed between 500 and 1,000 grams of fat a month, 42%

119

consumed between 1,001 and 1,500 grams of fat a month, 21% consumed between 1,501 and 2,000 grams of fat a month and 11% consumed between 2,001 and 3,000 grams of fat.

They reported their findings as follows: 'Consistent with our hypothesis, an effect of fat intake on survival time was reported in this study' and concluded that the 'estimated risk of death at any time increased 1.4 fold for every 1,000 gram in monthly fat intake'.

Exhibit F

Title

Dietary Factors and Breast Cancer Risk

Authors

Jay H. Lubin, Environmental Epidemiology Branch, National Cancer Institute, Bethesda, Maryland, U.S.A.; Patricia E. Burns, Cross Cancer Institute, Edmonton, Alberta, Canada; William J. Blot, Environmental Epidemiology Branch, National Cancer Institute, Bethesda, Maryland, U.S.A.; Regina G. Ziegler, Environmental Epidemiology Branch, National Cancer Institute, Bethesda, Maryland, U.S.A.; Alan W. Lees, Cross Cancer Institute, Edmonton, Alberta, Canada and Joseph F. Fraumeni, Jr., Environmental Epidemiology Branch, National Cancer Institute, Bethesda, Maryland, U.S.A.

Source

International Journal of Cancer

Date

1981

Report

These researchers questioned 577 women aged between 30 and 80 (all of whom had breast cancer) and 826 disease free women about their eating habits. They found that women who ate beef, pork and sweet desserts were significantly more likely to develop breast cancer than women who did not. They also found that women who fried with butter or margarine, as opposed to vegetable oils, and who used butter at the table were also more likely to develop breast cancer.

Exhibit G

Title

Role of Life-style and Dietary Habits in Risk of Cancer among Seventh-Day Adventists

Author

Roland L. Phillips, Department of Biostatistics and Epidemiology, Lorna Linda University School of Health, Lorna Linda, California, U.S.A.

Source

Cancer Research

Date

November 1975

Report

Seventh-Day Adventists neither drink alcohol nor smoke, most avoid the use of coffee, tea, hot condiments and spices and about half eat a vegetarian diet which includes dairy produce and eggs. In his summary the author noted that existing data on cancer mortality in Seventh-Day Adventists showed death rates that were 50% to 70% of the rates within the general population for most of the cancer sites that are unrelated to smoking or drinking alcohol. The author's studies showed statistically significant links between the eating of beef, lamb or a combined group of highly saturated fat foods and the development of colon cancer. 'It is quite clear,' he wrote, 'that these results are supportive of the hypothesis that beef, meat and saturated fat or fat in general are etiologically related to colon cancer.' He went on to say that: 'Green leafy vegetables that are quite high in fiber are negatively associated.'

The author concluded: 'Overall, the currently available evidence on cancer among Seventh-Day Adventists is consistent with the hypothesis that one or more components of the typical Adventist lifestyle account for a large portion of their apparent reduced risk of the types of cancer which are unrelated to cigarette smoking and alcohol consumption. Aside from abstinence from smoking and drinking, the most distinctive feature of the typical Adventist lifestyle is a unique diet whose principal feature is lacto-ovo-vegetarianism.' The author then added that other researchers had shown that the typical lacto-ovo-vegetarian diet contained about 25% less fat and 50% more fibre than the average non-vegetarian diet.

Exhibit H

Title

Diet as an Etiological Factor in the Development of Cancers of the Colon and Rectum

Author

Margaret A. Howell, National Cancer Institute, National Institutes of Health, Bethesda, Maryland, U.S.A.

Source

Journal of Chronic Diseases

Date

1975

Report

The author concludes: 'The evidence suggests that meat, particularly beef, is a food associated with the development of malignancies of the large bowel.'

Exhibit I

Title

Nutrient Intakes In Relation to Cancer Incidence in Hawaii

Authors

L. N. Kolonel, J. H. Hankin, J. Lee, S.Y Chu, A.M.Y Nomura and M. Ward Hinds — from the Epidemiology Program, Cancer Center of Hawaii, University of Hawaii, Honolulu, Hawaii, U.S.A.

Source

British Journal of Cancer

Date

1981

Report

For this study 4,657 adults from the five main ethnic groups in Hawaii (Caucasians, Japanese, Chinese, Hawaiians and Filipinos) were interviewed about their diets between the years 1977 and 1979. The researchers reported that: 'significant positive associations were found for six of the cancer sites: breast cancer with fat (saturated, unsaturated, animal and total) and protein (animal); corpus-uteri cancer with the same components as breast cancer, prostate cancer with fat (saturated, animal) and protein (animal, total), stomach cancer with fat (fish only) and protein (fish only), lung cancer with cholesterol and laryngeal cancer with cholesterol. The researchers also found significant negative associations between breast and corpus-uteri cancers and carbohydrate intake.

Exhibit J

Title

Environmental Factors of Cancer of the Colon and Rectum

Authors:

Ernest L. Wynder M.D., and Takao Shigematsu M.D., both from the Division of Environmental Cancerigenesis, Sloan Kettering Institute for Cancer Research, New York, U.S.A.

Source

Cancer

Date

September 1967

Report

The authors of this paper concluded: '...dietary factors appear to be associated with the etiology of cancer of the large bowel. The dietary pattern that may fit the distribution of cancer of the large bowel includes a high intake of fats. The effect of this pattern appears to be more marked for cancer of the colon than cancer of the rectum.' And they added: 'There is a statistically significant association of obesity to cancer of the large bowel from the cecum to the sigmoid colon in men.'

Exhibit K

Title

Epidemiological Correlations between Diet and Cancer Frequency

Author

Pelayo Correa, Louisiana State University Medical Center, New Orleans, Louisiana, U.S.A.

Source

Cancer Research

Date

September 1981

Report

The author stated that: 'Strong and consistent correlations are reported between death rates of cancers of the colon and breast and the per capita consumption of total fat and of nutrients derived from animal sources, especially beef, pork, eggs and milk. Similar but less consistent correlations have been reported with cancers of the prostate, ovary and endometrium.' The author also reported that: 'Negative correlations of colon cancer rates and vegetable consumption are reported ... Epidemiological data are consistent with the hypothesis that excessive beef and low vegetable consumption are causally related to colon cancer.' The author explained the link between the foods linked to cancer and the development of cancer by stating that 'these fooditems probably do not have a direct carcinogenic role but rather provide a microenvironment favourable to the actions of carcinogens.'

Exhibit L

Title

Food Consumption and Cancer of the Colon and Rectum in North-Eastern Italy

Authors

Ettore Bidoli, Epidemiology Unit, Aviano Cancer Center, Via Pedemontana Occ, Aviano, Italy; Silvia Franceschi, Epidemiology Unit, Aviano Cancer Center, Via Pedemontana Occ, Aviano, Italy and European Cancer Prevention Organisation, Epidemiology and Cancer Working Group, Brussels, Belgium; Renata Talamini, Epidemiology Unit, Aviano Cancer Center, Via Pedemontana Occ, Aviano, Italy; Salvatore Barra, Epidemiology Unit, Aviano Cancer Center, Via Pedemontana Occ, Aviano, Italy; and Carlo La Vecchia, Mario Negri Institute for Pharmacological Research, Via Eiritrea,

Milan, Italy and Institute of Social and Preventive Medicine, University of Lausanne, Lausanne, Switzerland

Source

International Journal of Cancer

Date

1992

Report

The authors studied 123 patients with colon cancer, 125 patients with rectal cancer and 699 patients with no cancer. They concluded: '...the present study gives support for a protective effect associated with a fiber rich or vegetable rich diet, while it indicates that frequent consumption of refined starchy foods, eggs and fat rich foods such as cheese and red meat is a risk factor for colorectal cancer.' The authors found that a high consumption of margarine 'exerted a significant protection against cancer of the colon' and that 'high consumption of carrots, spinach, whole grain bread and pasta' reduced the risk of rectal cancer.

Exhibit M

Title

Diet and Lung Cancer in California Seventh-Day Adventists

Authors

Gary E. Fraser, Center for Health Research, Lorna Linda University, Lorna Linda, California, U.S.A., W. Lawrence Beeson, Center for Health Research, Lorna Linda University, Lorna Linda, California, U.S.A. and Roland L. Phillips, Lorna Linda University, Lorna Linda, California, U.S.A.

Source

American Journal of Epidemiology

Date

1991

Report

The authors reported that: 'fruit consumption was the dietary constituent that showed a strong, statistically significant protective association with lung cancer...'

Exhibit N

Title

Dietary Habits and Past Medical History as Related to Fatal Pancreas Cancer Risk Among Adventists

Authors

Paul K. Mills Ph.D., W. Lawrence Beeson, M.S.P.H., David E. Abbey Ph.D., Gary E. Fraser M.D., Ph.D., and Roland L. Phillips M.D., DrPH, from the Department of Preventive Medicine, School of Medicine, Lorna Linda University, Lorna Linda, California, U.S.A.

Source

Cancer

Date

1988

Report

The authors began by pointing out that the foods and/or nutrients which had been suggested to be associated with an increased risk of cancer of the prostate included 'total fat intake, eggs, animal protein, sugar, meat, coffee and butter' whereas the consumption of 'raw fruits and vegetables' had been 'consistently associated with decreased risk'. In this study the authors found that there was strong evidence that 'increasing consumption of vegetarian protein products, beans, lentils and peas as well as dried fruit' helped to protect against cancer of the pancreas.

Exhibit O

Title

Increasing use of soyfoods and their potential role in cancer prevention

Authors

Mark Messina Ph.D, Diet and Cancer Branch, Division of Cancer Prevention and Control, National Cancer Institute, Bethesda, U.S.A. Virginia Messina PhD, RD., Washington, U.S.A.

Source

Journal American Diet Association

Date

July 1991

Report

Most of the soya beans produced are used as animal feed but evidence has been accumulating that soybeans can prevent cancer. The authors of this report state that: 'Soybeans contain, in relatively high concentrations, several compounds with demonstrated anticarcinogenic activity.'

Exhibit P

Title

Dietary Prevention of Breast Cancer

Authors

David P. Rose and Jeanne M. Connolly, Division of Nutrition and Endocrinology, American Health Foundation, Valhalla, New York, U.S.A.

Source

Med.Oncol & Tumour Pharmacother.

Date

1990

Report

A review of the epidemiological and experimental data suggests that dietary modification does have a place in breast cancer prevention,' say the authors. 'Based on present evidence, a dietary approach to breast cancer prevention should include weight control, when indicated, a reduction in dietary fat in-take to approximately 20% total intake, and an increase in fiber consumption to 25-30 grams a day.'

Exhibit Q

Title

Shift From a Mixed Diet to a Lactovegetarian Diet: Influence on Some Cancer-Associated Intestinal Bacterial Enzyme Activities

Authors

Gunnar K. Johansson, Ludmila Ottova and Jan-Ake Gustafsson (the authors are affiliated with the Department of Medical Nutrution, Karolinska Institute, Huddinge University Hospital, Huddinge, Sweden).

Source

Nutr. Cancer

Date

1990

Report

The authors of this paper conclude: '...the results in this paper indicate that a change from a mixed diet to a lactovegetariandiet leads to a decrease in certain enzyme activities proposed to be risk factors for colon cancer.'

Exhibit R

Title

Nutritional Approach to Oesophageal Cancer in Scotland

Author

Valda M Craddock, M.R.C. Toxicology Unit, Carshalton, Surrey, U.K.

Source

The Lancet

Date

24th January 1987

Report

This publication took the form of a letter. The author began by pointing out that oesophageal cancer has a sharply defined geographical distribution in Britain — with many sufferers being in the north-west of Scotland where the consumption of green vegetables is believed to be low.

The author also pointed out that oesophageal cancer is also very common in areas of China, in Iran, around the Caspian Sea and in parts of South Africa and adds that in all these regions the diet is low in fresh fruit and green vegetables — and the micronutrients they contain. A consistent finding from studies around the world of diet in relation to cancer is that consumption of fresh green vegetables is negatively associated with cancer,' writes the author. 'Deaths in women from this exceptionally distressing malignant disease total around 2,000 per year. Early diagnosis is not yet possible and treatment is unsatisfactory. Prevention, however, may be relatively easy.' The author also adds that the incidence of oesophageal cancer in Britain has almost doubled since 1970 and that 'there are epidemiological and experimental grounds for intervention studies which might lead to effective preventive measures, but nothing is being done.'

Exhibit S

Title

Cohort Study of Diet, Lifestyle and Prostate Cancer in Adventist Men

Authors

Paul K. Mills, Ph.D, MPH; W. Lawrence Beeson, MSPH; Roland L. Phillips, M.D. DrPH, and Gary E. Fraser M.D., Ph.D; from the Department of Preventive Medicine, Lorna Linda University School of Medicine, Lorna Linda, California, U.S.A.

Source

Cancer

Date

1989

Report

For this study the authors evaluated dietary and lifestyle characteristics of approximately 14,000 Seventh-Day Adventist men. The men completed a detailed lifestyle questionnaire in 1976 and were monitored for cancer incidence until the end of 1982. The authors concluded that: 'increasing consumption of beans, lentils and peas, tomatoes, raisin, dates and other dried fruit were all associated with significantly decreased prostate cancer risk.'

Exhibit T

Title

A Prospective Study of Dietary Fat and Risk of Prostate Cancer

Authors

Edward Giovannucci, Channing Laboratory, Department of Medicine, Harvard Medical School and Brigham and Women's Hospital, Boston, Mass, U.S.A.; Eric B. Rimm, Department of Epidemiology, Harvard School of Public Health, Boston, U.S.A.; Graham A. Colditz, Channing Laboratory, Department of Medicine,

Harvard Medical School and Brigham and Women's Hospital, Department of Epidemiology, Harvard School of Public Health, Boston, U.S.A.; Meir J. Stampfer, Channing Laboratory,Department of Medicine, Harvard Medical School and Brigham and Women's Hospital, Department of Epidemiology, Harvard School of Public Health, Boston, U.S.A.; Alberto Ascherio, Department of Nutrition, Harvard School of Public Health, Boston, U.S.A.; Chris C. Chute, Department of Health Sciences Research, Mayo Medical School, Rochester, Minn., U.S.A.; Walter C. Willett, Channing Laboratory, Department of Medicine, Harvard Medical School and Brigham and Women's Hospital, Department of Epidemiology and Department of Nutrition, Harvard School of Public Health, Boston, U.S.A.

Source

Journal of the National Cancer Institute

Date

October 6th 1993

Report

The authors pointed out that: 'The strong correlation between national consumption of fat and national rate of mortality from prostate cancer has raised the hypothesis that dietary fat increases the risk of this malignancy.' By studying information relating to 51,529 American men between the ages of 40 and 75 and sending follow up questionnaires to the men in 1988 and 1990 they examined the relationship of fat consumption to the incidence of advanced prostate cancer and to the total incidence of prostate cancer.

The authors found that 'total fat consumption was directly related to risk of advanced prostate cancer' and that 'this association was due primarily to animal fat... but not vegetable fat. Red meat represented the food group with the strongest positive association with advanced cancer.'

The authors concluded that: 'The results support the hypothesis that animal fat, especially fat from red meat, is associated with an elevated risk of advanced prostate cancer.' They also noted that: 'These findings support recommendations to lower intake of meat to reduce the risk of prostate cancer.'

Exhibit U

Title

Risk of death from cancer and ischaemic heart disease in meat and non-meat eaters

Authors

Margaret Thorogood, senior research fellow, Department of Public Health and Policy, London School of Hygiene and Tropical Medicine, London, UK; Jim Mann, professor, Department of Human Nutrition, University of Otago, Dunedin, New Zealand; Paul Appleby, research officer, Department of Public Health and Primary Care, University of Oxford, Oxford, U.K.; Klim McPherson, professor, Department of Public Health and Policy, London School of Hygiene and Tropical Medicine, London, U.K.

Source

British Medical Journal

Date

25th June 1994

Report

The aim of this research was to investigate the health consequences of a vegetarian diet by examining the twelve year mortality of vegetarians and meat eaters. The researchers reported: 'These data confirm the findings of previous studies that have shown a reduction in all cause, cancer and cardiovascular mortality among people who do not eat meat.'

The researchers showed a 'roughly 40% reduction in mortality from cancer in vegetarians and fish eaters compared with meat eaters' and also added that 'the fact that total mortality was about 20% lower in the non-meat eating group than the meat eaters is perhaps of greatest clinical importance.'

Exhibit V

Title

Risk Factors for Renal-Cell Cancer in Shanghai, China **Authors**

Joseph K. McLaughlin, National Cancer Institute, Division of Cancer Etiology, Epidemiology and Biostatistics Program, Bethesda, MD, U.S.A; Yu-Tang Gao, Shanghai Cancer Institute, Department of Epidemiology, Shanghai, People's Republic of China; Ru-Nie Gao, Shanghai Cancer Institute, Department of Epidemiology, Shanghai, People's Republic of China; Wei Zheng, National Cancer Institute, Division of Cancer Etiology, Epidemiology and Biostatistics Program, Bethesda, MD, U.S.A; Bu-Tianji, Shanghai Cancer Institute, Department of Epidemiology, Shanghai, People's Republic of China; William J. Blot, National Cancer Institute, Division of Cancer Etiology, Epidemiology and Biostatistics Program, Bethesda, MD, U.S.A; and Joseph F. Fraumeni Jr, National Cancer Institute, Division of Cancer Etiology, Epidemiology and Biostatistics Program, Bethesda, MD, U.S.A.

Source

International Journal of Cancer

Date

1992

Report

The authors studied 154 patients with renal cell cancer and 157 controls. They reported: 'Elevated risks were observed for cigarette smoking...and for increasing categories of body weight and meat consumption, while reduced risks were seen for increasing categories of fruit and vegetable intake. An increase was also observed for regular use of phenacetin containing analgesics.' The authors also noted that these findings were 'consistent with earlier studies in Western countries and indicate that many of the same etiologic factors for renal cell cancer operate in low and high risk societies.'

Exhibit W
Title
Shift from a mixed to a lactovegetarian diet: influence on acid lipids in fecal water — a potential risk factor for colon cancer
Authors
Ulrika Geltner Allinger, Gunnar K. Johansson, Jan-Ake Gustafsson and Joseph J. Rafter; from the Department of Medical Nutrition, Karolinska Institute, Huddinge University Hospital, Huddinge, Sweden
Source
The American Journal of Clinical Nutrition
Date
1989
Report
The authors concluded that: 'the consumption of a lactovegetarian diet may reduce certain risk factors of potential significance in colon carcinogenesis.'

Exhibit X
Title
NCI dietary guidelines: rationale
Authors

Ritva R. Butrum Ph.D., Carolyn K. Clifford Ph.D., and Elaine Lanza Ph.D from the Division of Cancer Prevention and Control, National Cancer Institute, National Institutes of Health, Bethesda, MD, US.A

Source

The American Journal of Clinical Nutrition

Date

1988

Report

The authors report that in 1986 it was estimated that 930,000 Americans would develop cancer and that 472,000 individuals would die of their cancer.

The National Cancer Institute (the NCI), which aims to reduce cancer incidence, morbidity and mortality, 'believes that the potential for dietary changes to reduce the risk of cancer is considerable and that the existing scientific data provide evidence that is sufficiently consistent to warrant prudent interim dietary guidelines that will promote good health and reduce the risk of some types of cancer.'

The NCI suggests reducing fat intake, increasing fibre intake, including a variety of fruits and vegetables in the daily diet, avoiding obesity, consuming alcoholic beverages in moderation if at all and minimising the consumption of salt cured, salt pickled and smoked foods. The NCI believes that if these guidelines were followed there would be a 50% reduction in cancer of the colon and rectum, a 25% reduction in breast cancer and a 15% reduction in cancers of the prostate, endometrium and gallbladder.

Exhibit Y

Title

Shifting from a Conventional Diet to an Uncooked Vegan Diet Reversibly Alters Fecal Hydrolytic Activities in Humans

Authors

Wen Hua Ling and Osmo Hanninen from the Department of Physiology, University of Kuopio, Kuopio, Finland

Source

Journal of Nutrition

Date

1992

Report

The authors conclude that an 'uncooked extreme vegan diet causes a decrease in bacterial enzymes and certain toxic products that have been implicated in colon cancer risk.'

Exhibit Z

Title

Association between dietary changes and mortality rates: Israel 1949 to 1977; a trend-free regression model

Author

Aviva Palgi Ph.D., Instructor in Nutrition, Harvard Medical School, Nutrition/Metabolism Laboratory, New England Deaconess Hospital, United States of America

Source

The American Journal of Clinical Nutrition

Date

August 1981

Report

The author investigated the statistical effect of 'changes in food consumption of the Israeli population during 1949 to 1977 on concurrent mortality rates from cancer, heart disease, peptic ulcer, and diabetes mellitus'.

The author reported that: 'All the investigated mortality rates were in statistically significant positive association with increasing total fat consumption. Mortality rates of ischemic heart disease as well as of hypertensive and cerebrovascular disease were in positive association with both plant fat and animal fat. These findings suggest that reduced total fat intake may prove to reduce the investigated mortality rates.'

Note 1

Where I have included medical or scientific qualifications alongside the names of researchers it is because these were published on the scientific papers concerned. Where no qualifications are listed it is because no qualifications were listed on the journal articles I have quoted.

Note 2

In January 1986 the *Journal of Occupational Medicine* published a paper entitled *Cancer Mortality Among White Males in the Meat Industry*. The paper was written by Eric S. Johnson M.B., B.S.; H. R. Fischman D.VM.; Genevieve M. Martanoski M.D.; and E. Diamond Ph.D. from the Department of Epidemiology, The Johns Hopkins University School of Hygiene and Public Health, Baltimore, United States of America. The authors studied 13,844 members of a meat cutter's union from July 1949 to December 1980 'to examine cancer occurrence in the meat industry'. They reported that a 'statistically significant proportional mortality ratio of 2.9 was obtained for Hodgkin's disease among abattoir workers' and that 'the results suggest that the excess risk of death from Hodgkin's disease in abattoir workers may be associated with the slaughtering activity'.

They also found that meat packing plant workers were more likely to develop bone cancer, cancer of the buccal cavity and pharynx and lung cancer than workers in other industries.

I report this paper because although it does not show a direct link between cancer and the eating of meat as a food it does pose an important question: if human beings can get cancer merely by handling meat why on earth should there be any surprise that human beings can get cancer from eating meat? The authors of this paper also named viruses which naturally cause cancer in cattle and chickens and pointed out that these viruses are present not only in diseased but also in healthy cattle and chickens destined for human consumption. 'Evidence suggests that consumers of meat and unpasteurized milk may be exposed to these viruses. It would appear, therefore, that these viruses present a potentially serious public health problem.' Other researchers have made similar discoveries about a link between the meat industry and the development of cancer. A study of 300,000 adult white males in Washington State in the United States of America showed a 'statistically significant elevated risk of death from cancer of the buccal cavity and pharynx among butchers and meat cutters'.

CHAPTER TWELVE

FOODS TO AVOID — AND FOODS TO EAT — TO CUT YOUR CANCER RISK

However careful you are to avoid cancer-inducing chemicals, cancer cells will occasionally develop inside your body Most of the time those cancer cells are dealt with speedily and effectively by your body's defence systems. White blood cells find and destroy cancer cells in just the same way that they find and destroy bacteria.

Your body's natural immune system (and its ability to deal with cancer) will be damaged if you eat the wrong sort of foods — and will be aided and improved if you eat the right foods. Fatty foods will weaken your immune system and make your body less capable of fighting off those occasional cancer cells. When researchers studied the blood of human volunteers they found that a low fat diet greatly improved the activity of the body's natural killer cells.

Incidentally, it has been shown that as far as the body's immune system is concerned vegetable fats are just as bad as animal fats. You will protect your heart by reducing your animal fat consumption but in order to protect yourself against cancer you need to reduce your entire fat consumption — and that includes vegetable oils.

Vegetarians have more than double the cancer cell destroying capability of non-vegetarians. But this is not entirely due to the low fat content of a vegetarian diet. It is probably also due to the fact that vegetarians consume fewer toxic chemicals and no animal proteins.

And vegetarians have another advantage too: the ability of the human body's natural killer cells to do their work is improved by substances such as beta-carotene which are found in considerable quantities in vegetables. (One survey of meat eaters showed that many could neither name nor describe any green vegetables.)

Foods to avoid

FATTY FOODS IN GENERAL

The average diet still contains 40% fat. Many official recommendations are still only encouraging a reduction in fat intake to around 30% of the diet — despite evidence showing that a reduction to somewhere between 10% and 20% would make far more sense. Fat was the first dietary constituent to be linked with cancer and there is now probably more evidence damning fat than any other foodstuff. According to the National Academy of Sciences report *Diet, Nutrition and Cancer* (published by the National Academy Press in Washington DC, US in 1982) there were at least six international studies published in the 1970s which showed a direct association between the amount of fat eaten and breast cancer incidence or mortality. In addition a state by state study published within the US showed a significant direct correlation between fat intake and breast cancer mortality rates.

'Japanese women have the lowest breast cancer rate in the world',' says Dr Oliver Alabaster, Director of the Institute for Disease Prevention at the George Washington University Medical Center, quoted in *The Power of your Plate,* by Dr Neal D Barnard. 'Many Japanese women have migrated to Hawaii andthe US mainland. While marrying within their own community and keeping the population relatively unchanged genetically, they shifted their diet towards a more Western, higher fat diet and their breast cancer rate steadily climbed. A few decades ago the Japanese diet contained only around 10% fat — today the average Japanese diet contains about 25% fat. Within one generation it approximated that of

Caucasian women living around them. This is very dramatic evidence that cancer is mainly environmentally induced, rather than genetically inherited.'

Peter Greenwald, Director of Cancer Prevention and Control of the National Cancer Institute in the United States of America also says that there is a great deal of evidence that fat increases cancer risk and points out that the differences in breast cancer rates in different countries cannot be due to other factors such as stress, pollution or industrialisation since there are highly industrialised countries such as Japan where stress and pollution are as high as the US or Europe but where colon and breast cancer rates are low.

Since the mid 1970s there has been strong evidence to show a link between a high fat intake and prostate cancer. The National Academy of Sciences reports that an American study showed a correlation between a high fat intake and a high risk for prostate cancer. Studies in 41 countries have shown a high correlation between mortality from prostate cancer and intake of fats, milk and meats (especially beef). A ten year Japanese study involving 122,261 men aged 40 or older showed 'an inverse association between daily intake of green and yellow vegetables and mortality from prostate cancer'. Another study showed that vegetarian men were less likely to develop prostate cancer.

Other studies also confirm this link. In 1993 a study of 47,855 men, reported in the *Medical Research Modernization Committee Report* revealed that those men who had high fat diets had a relative risk of 1.79 for advanced prostate cancer compared to those on a low fat diet. The investigators found that 'most animal fats were associated with advanced prostate cancer, but fats from vegetables, dairy products (except butter) and fish were not.'

The National Academy of Sciences reports that: 'other reproductive organs for which there have been associations between dietary fat and cancer include the testes, corpus uteri, and ovary'.

There is also a considerable amount of published evidence available to show that there is a firm association between dietary fat and gastrointestinal tract cancer. Some researchers have shown a link between dietary fat and cancer of the pancreas, and others have shown a link between fat and stomach cancer. Researchers have also accumulated strong evidence confirming a correlation between dietary fat and large bowel cancer (cancers of the colon and rectum).

The National Academy of Sciences reports that: 'In general, it is not possible to identify specific components of fat as being clearly responsible for the observed effects, although total fat and saturated fat have been associated most frequently.'

With all this evidence available directly from observations of human patients it is exceedingly difficult to see why such a large proportion of the cancer industry's budget is spent on performing experiments on animals.

Although the evidence showing that fat causes cancer is totally convincing (a United States Surgeon General has advised US citizens that 'a comparison of populations indicates that death rates for cancers of the breast, colon and prostate are directly proportional to estimated dietary fat intakes') there is still a considerable amount of doubt about the mechanism whereby fat causes cancer.

One theory is that carcinogenic chemicals simply dissolve and accumulate in fatty tissues. If this is the case then people who eat animal fats will suffer twice for the chances are high that the fat they are eating already contains dissolved carcinogens. Another possibility is that fat may encourage the development of cancer by affecting the activity of sex hormones. Vegetarian and low fat diets reduce the levels of circulating female sex hormones such as oestradiol. Sex hormones are known to help promote the development of breast cancer and cancer of the reproductive organs (such as uterus and ovary in women and the prostate in men).

Despite the lack of clear evidence about exactly how fat causes cancer the final message is quite clear — to reduce your cancer risk you should make a real effort to cut back your fat intake — and that includes cutting out vegetable fats too. You should not make the mistake of assuming that you can avoid or cut down your fat intake noticeably by living on a diet of chicken and fish. Although it is widely believed that both fish and chicken are low in fat the truth is that even skinless white meat from a chicken is 23% fat while most fish contain between 20 to 30% fat and some are much higher — mackerel, for example, contains over 50% fat. The only truly low fat diet is a diet which is mainly composed of vegetables, fruits, and whole grain cereals. Rice contains only about 1% fat and no plant foods contain any cholesterol (although frying potatoes and turning them into chips can add a lot of fat).

If you ignore this message then you are making a clear and conscious choice to accept a high cancer risk as the price for your high fat diet.

MEAT AND ANIMAL PRODUCTS

Numerous researchers have linked protein with cancers of the breast, prostate, endometrium (lining of the uterus), colon and rectum, pancreas and kidney. And the type of protein which is most likely to cause cancer is protein obtained from meat.

The United States Surgeon General's Report Nutrition and Health said: 'In one international correlational study, for example, a positive association was observed between total protein and animal protein and breast, colon, prostate, renal and endometrial cancers (Armstrong and Doll 1975). Similarly, a migrant study indicated an association between meat consumption and cancer of the breast and colon (Kolonel 1987).'

The Surgeon General also reported that: 'Studies have also found an association between breast cancer and meat intake (Lubin et al 1981) and an association of meat, especially beef, with large bowel cancer among Japanese (Haenszel et al 1973)...'

One possible reason for the meat-cancer link may be the fact that chemicals such as DDT tend to accumulate in animal tissues — and may be found in animal tissues years after their usage has been controlled or stopped. Whether it is the chemicals in animal protein which cause cancer is, however, a question of rather theoretical interest: the important point is that meat causes cancer.

There is evidence to show that Japanese women who eat meat daily have more than eight times the risk of breast cancer compared to poorer women who rarely consume meat.

There have also been several reports showing a high correlation between meat (an important source of dietary fat, especially saturated fat) and colon cancer. Beef has been specifically named as one type of meat associated with colon cancer. Several studies have shown a relationship between the incidence of prostate cancer and the consumption of animal protein.

Because most people who eat a lot of meat usually also eat a great deal of fat (because meat often contains a lot of fat) it is difficult to know whether these links between meat and cancer are a result of the protein in the meat or the fat in the meat. It is also possible that the link between meat and cancer is a result of mutagens being formed during the cooking of meat. And some experts have pointed out that carcinogenic fat-soluble contaminants

145

such as drugs and pesticides may be the reason why meat causes cancer.

However, I regard the question of how meat causes cancer as being of largely theoretical interest. The important thingis that most of us need to eat less protein in general — and since there is a link between meat and cancer it seems pretty clear that cutting out meat is a sensible way to cut down protein.

DAIRY PRODUCTS

The consumption of milk and other dairy products is relatively new in human history. And it is only in the 'highly developed' and 'Westernised' world that milk drinking is considered essential or even normal.

Milk drinking (and the consumption of other dairy products) has developed because farmers and marketing experts have created the products and not because consuming these products is normal, essential or healthy. Babies need their mother's milk, taken direct from the breast, but no human beings need to drink dairy milk, or eat butter or cheese or other dairy products.

It is almost certainly the fat in dairy products which makes them particularly dangerous. Inevitably, therefore, some dairy products are more dangerous than others. Butter and cream and high fat cheeses are far more likely to cause problems than are low fat yoghurt, low fat cheese or skimmed milk.

But it isn't only the fat in dairy products which causes problems. There has for some years been accumulating evidence to suggest that dairy products can cause a wide variety of illnesses and there is now also some evidence to suggest that dairy products may be a contributory factor in the development of cancer of the ovary. The problem is, it seems, that a sugar in milk called lactose is broken down within the body to produce another sugar called galactose — which is then, in turn, broken down again. But if the consumption of dairy produce exceeds the body's ability to break down galactose this sugar may accumulate in the blood — and have an effect on the ovaries. Drinking low or non-fat milk won't help this particular problem because the problem is caused by a sugar not fat.

ALCOHOL

It has been known for some years that there is an association between alcohol abuse and cancer. In 1937, in France, it was noted that 95% of patients with oesophageal cancer were alcohol abusers. Another French study, published in the 1960s and involving 4,000 patients, showed a significant correlation between alcohol consumption and cancers of the tongue, hypopharynx and larynx. In 1964 the World Health Organisation concluded that: 'excessive consumption of alcoholic beverages was associated with cancer of the mouth, larynx and oesophagus'. A Finnish study, published in 1974, showed that chronic alcoholics were more likely to develop cancers of the pharynx, oesophagus and lung.

Alcohol has also been linked with cancer of the stomach and cancer of the pancreas. In 1988 the United States Surgeon General reported that: 'Reviews of experimental and epidemiological data suggest an association between alcohol consumption and human cancer that is strongest for certain head and neck cancers.'

Smoking seems to make matters even worse and there is a synergistic carcinogenic relationship between alcohol and smoking tobacco: people who drink a good deal of alcohol and smoke tobacco are particularly likely to suffer from cancer of the mouth, larynx, oesophagus and respiratory tract.

You don't have to give up drinking alcohol completely in order to avoid or minimise this cancer risk. If you enjoy a glass of wine with a meal or a glass of whisky afterwards then that's fine. I myself am rather partial to a glass of malt whisky. But limit yourself to one or possibly two drinks a day at most.

FOOD ADDITIVES

Over 15,000 chemical substances are added to food as it is processed. Some of these chemicals are introduced deliberately (to add flavour, colour and consistency and so on) but many thousands of chemicals are added indirectly, either because they are used in food packaging or because they have been consumed by animals (as drugs or hormones) before finding their way into animal products.

Only a very small number of the substances added to foods have been tested for carcinogenicity and very few epidemiological studies have been conducted to find out whether or not there are any relationships between food additives and cancer incidence. At least one government has admitted that there are too many additives for them all to be fully tested. (The extent of the problem can be seen from the fact that any comprehensive testing programme would have to examine any possible synergistic activity between any combination of the many thousands of additives used.)

SMOKED, SALTED AND PICKLED FOODS

Substances which are potentially carcinogenic are produced in charred meat and fish because of changes in the proteins in those foods which occur when foods are cooked at very high temperatures.

Cooking foods over charcoal or smoking foods results in the food being covered with carcinogenic substances. In 1964 it was reported that beef grilled over a gas or charcoal fire contained polycyclic aromatic hydrocarbons (PAHs) produced from smoke generated by the dripping of fat from the meat onto the hot coals. Polycyclic aromatic hydrocarbons have also been found in a number of different types of smoked foods. Polycyclic aromatic hydrocarbons account for some of the potentially carcinogenic changes that occur in food during cooking.

The United States Surgeon General has reported that: 'International epidemiological evidence suggests that populations consuming diets high in salt-cured, salt-pickled, and smoked foods have a higher incidence of stomach and oesophageal cancers.'

The available evidence suggests that it is wisest to avoidfood which has been salt-cured, salt-pickled, smoked or cooked on a barbecue.

Foods to eat

FIBRE

Until relatively recently fibre was regarded as an entirely inert substance — an unnecessary 'filler' that simply took up space in food, on the plate and in your stomach. There were even many experts who regarded fibre as a nuisance — something to be removed from food whenever possible. It was argued that because of its bulky presence fibre might interfere with the absorption of essential minerals.

The research work of Dr Denis Burkitt and other doctors changed that point of view for ever. It is now clear that fibre passes through the small intestines without being digested but that it removes harmful substances and helps to speed up the passage of food through the intestinal tract.

Once it had been recognised that people who ate a 'primitive diet' (rich in complex carbohydrates such as fibre) were less likely to suffer from a range of disorders, including bowel cancer, the popularity of fibre began to rise.

Burkitt noted that colorectal cancer (cancers of the colon and rectum) is rare among primitive people who eat unrefined foods.

Inevitably, perhaps, the food industry's immediate, knee jerk response to this discovery was to start selling consumers bran and fibre supplements. Instead of encouraging people to buy more natural foods, full of natural fibre, the massive, international industry continued to sell packaged foods from which the fibre had been removed — but added a new range of foods which had been artificially enriched with fibre and many new varieties of fibre supplements. It was a trick of stupefying audacity, but it worked: all around the globe, in so called developed countries, people who regarded themselves as educatedand intelligent consumers sought to balance their fibre deprived diets by purchasing and swallowing these artificial fibre supplements. Having paid the food industry to take the essential fibre out of their food they then paid the industry a second time to buy the fibre back.

Dietary fibre usually includes indigestible carbohydrates and carbohydrate like food components such as cellulose, lignin, hemicellulose, pentosans, gums and pectins — all of which provide bulk. The foods that usually provide fibre are vegetables, fruits and whole grain cereals.

Researchers are still trying to decide whether fibre helps prevent cancer directly or whether it works by helping to rid the body of carcinogenic substances. Fibre can dilute the carcinogens present in the large bowel; it can influence the composition and activity of the flora living in the intestine; it can affect the production of carcinogenic substances and it can speed up the rate at which food passes through the bowel (thereby reducing the amount of time that carcinogens are in contact with bowel tissue). Fibre seems to affect cholesterol metabolism and it is also believed to reduce the levels of hormones which may lead to the development of cancer.

There is evidence that fibre helps to balance the cancer producing effect of fat in the diet. When you eat a fatty meal the gallbladder produces bile acids which flow into the intestine. The job of the bile acids is to help with the absorption of the fat in your meal. Bacteria which already exist within the intestine turn the bile acids into substances called secondary bile acids which are believed to promote the development of cancer. Fibre helps by having an effect on the bacteria in the intestine and, because it has a 'blotting paper' effect, by absorbing the bile acids. Because fibre takes up a lot of space it also dilutes the effect of the potentially harmful substances. In addition fibre is believed to delay the onset of menstruation in young girls. Girls who are brought up on a primitive, fibre-rich diet start to menstruate several years later than girls who are broughtup on a typical, fat-rich, fibre-poor 'Western' diet. This is important because there is also evidence to show that the risk of breast cancer goes up as the onset of menstruation comes down. Just how fibre has all these effects is still the subject of some discussion although it has been suggested that specific components of fibre are more likely than fibre *per se* to be responsible for protecting humans against cancer.

As far as you and I are concerned, however, I believe that all this theory and all this research is only of academic value. The important thing to know is that your diet should contain a plentiful supply of natural fibre. You can get fibre from vegetables and beans and whole wheat bread, brown rice and cereals. Fibre is lost from refined grains and no foods made from dead animals contain fibre.

151

VEGETABLES AND FRUIT

One advantage of eating more vegetable products is undoubtedly the fact that by so doing you will inevitably eat few animal products — foodstuffs which are known to cause cancer. But fruit and vegetables have positive values too.

Vegetables and fruit also contain fibre — and some vegetables (cruciferous vegetables — cabbage, cauliflower, Brussels sprouts and broccoli) contain constituents (such as indoles and isothiocyanates) which are believed to have an anti-cancer effect.

A large number of scientific studies have shown that an individual's risk of developing cancer (particularly cancer of the gastro-intestinal tract — including the stomach and the large bowel) goes down if he eats more vegetables. No one really knows for certain why this is — but once again the exact mechanism by which the consumption of vegetables protects against the development of cancer is much less important than the existence of the relationship.

In 1972 it was found that the consumption of raw vegetables, including coleslaw and red cabbage seemed to protect against stomach cancer. In 1975 it was found that the consumption of fibre rich foods such as cabbage protected against colon cancer. In 1978 it was reported that individuals who frequently ate raw vegetables (especially cabbage, brussels sprouts and broccoli) were less likely to develop cancer of the colon.

Garlic and onions contain large quantities of a chemical which seems to have anti-cancer properties. People who eat large quantities of garlic and onions have less than half the risk of stomach cancer of people who either don't eat these vegetables at all or who eat them in very small quantities.

There are many other substances found in vegetables and fruits which seem to help prevent cancer. Phenols, flavones, protease inhibitors, glutathione and beta-sitosterol are just a few of the natural chemicals found in vegetables and fruits which seem to have an anti-cancer effect. And there is evidence to suggest that many vegetables and fruits contain antimutagens which help protect cells against the activity of mutagens — substances which damage a cell's DNA and can turn an ordinary cell into a cancerous cell.

There have been many attempts to explain the protective effects of vegetables but I believe the important thing is that the inverse relationship between these vegetables and the development of cancer (that is the fact that those who eat these vegetables are less likely to develop cancer) has been clearly and indisputably established.

In 1982 the American National Academy of Sciences concluded that there is sufficient epidemiological evidence to suggest that consumption of certain vegetables, especially carotene rich (i.e. dark green and deep yellow) vegetables and cruciferous vegetables (e.g. cabbage, broccoli, cauliflower and Brussels sprouts) is associated with a reduction in the incidence of cancer at several sites in humans.

WHOLE GRAINS

Whole grains (rice, oats, wheat, barley etc. which have not been processed and had part of the 'goodness' removed) contain fibre, vitamin E and selenium — all of which can help reduce your risk of developing cancer.

VITAMINS AND MINERALS

For the last two decades there has been a considerable amount of discussion about the value of vitamins (particularly vitamins A and C) in the prevention — and even treatment — of cancer. In vitamin A it is the beta-carotene content which is believed to have the protective quality. (A large body of evidence suggests that foods

153

high in vitamin A and carotenoids are protective against a variety of epithelial cancers', said the US Surgeon General.)

Researchers have found that people who eat a diet which is low in vitamin A tend to be more likely to suffer from cancers of the lung, larynx, bladder, oesophagus, stomach, colon, rectum and prostate.

With vitamin C researchers have again found that this vitamin may lower the risk of cancer; in particular, it seems to lower the risk of cancer of the oesophagus and stomach.

Some of those who advocate meat eating claim that vegetarians are likely to have a diet which is deficient in iron. This is nonsense. A good, well-balanced vegetarian diet will contain plenty of iron. Indeed, there is now evidence to suggest that too much iron in the blood (a problem which can occur among meat eaters) increases the chances of cancer developing. When iron has been absorbed the body stores it. In many Westernised countries iron 'overload' is thought to be more common than iron deficiency. According to the American Physicians Committee for Responsible Medicine 'higher amounts of iron in the blood mean a higher cancer risk.' It also appears that iron that comes from animal sources is more likely to cause heart disease.

Zinc is another mineral which is believed to have some beneficial effects on cancer risk. Dr Melvyn R. Werbach's excellent source book *Nutritional Influences on Illness* lists three scientific papers which have shown that there may be a link betweena low zinc intake and prostate cancer. One paper showed that serum levels in prostatic cancer are low when compared to patients who have benign prostatic hypertrophy. A second paper showed that prostatic tissue levels of zinc are low in prostatic cancer compared to normal men. And a third paper showed that prostatic tissue levels are low in prostatic cancer compared to patients with prostatic hyperplasia.

Sadly, there still seems to be insufficient evidence available for me to offer solid guidelines on the subject of zinc and prostate cancer. It seems a pity that the cancer industry (the recipient of billions of dollars in charitable contributions) has not done more work into this possible link. Prostate cancer is, of course, one of the major killers of men.

Zinc is present in rice, corn and oats, spinach, peas and potatoes and so a good, well-balanced vegetarian diet should provide a plentiful supply. It is possible that too much zinc (as with most things) may cause damage.

Finally, it is worth pointing out that human experiments have shown that your body can repair the DNA which has been damaged by free radicals if it receives a plentiful supply of folic acid — one of the vitamin B complex of vitamins. Your body will receive the folic acid it needs if you eat a diet which is rich in dark green, leafy vegetables, fruits, dried peas, beans and wheat germ.

Foods which contain anti-oxidants (beta carotene, vitamin C, vitamin E):

* Apple
* Broccoli
* Brussels sprouts
* Cauliflower
* Chick peas
* Corn
* Grapefruit
* Orange
* Pineapple

* Brown rice
* Soya beans
* Spinach
* Strawberries
* Sweet Potato

Foods which contain folic acid

* Asparagus
* Baked beans
* Black beans
* Black eyed peas
* Broccoli
* Brussels sprouts
* Chick peas
* Kidney beans
* Lentils
* Soya beans
* Spinach

CHAPTER THIRTEEN

OTHER COMMON DISEASES — AND THEIR RELATIONSHIP TO WHAT YOU EAT

The diet you choose to eat will determine what illnesses you suffer from and how healthy you are. Most of us eat too much fat, too much meat, too much sugar and far too little fresh fruit, fresh vegetables and fibre. The list of diseases known to be associated with the food we eat grows longer every year and now includes an enormous variety of problems, ranging from asthma to cancer and heart disease to varicose veins.

Note

If you are suffering from any of the medical problems listed below do talk to your doctor before changing your eating habits. It is possible that if you change your eating habits your need for medical help may change too. For example, if you suffer from high blood pressure and normally take tablets to control your condition, changing your diet may reduce your need for medication.

Acne

Several scientific studies have shown that there are powerful links between eating habits and acne — one of the commonest, most troublesome and most embarrassing of all skin disorders. Doctors have shown that Eskimos who change to a Western diet develop more acne than Eskimos who remain faithful to their traditional, more natural diet which contains far less sugar. It has also been shown that there is less acne among black people living in Kenya and Zambia and surviving on a traditional diet than there is among black people of similar origins living in America — one of the main differences between the two groups is, of course, the diet that they eat. It is clear from the evidence which is now available that you can help clear up acne by eating less fat and less sugar and by eating more fibre.

Allergies

Asthma, dermatitis, eczema, hay fever and rhinitis are all much more common now than they were a few decades ago. Two generations ago eczema affected two people out of every thousand. Today the same disorder affects six times as many people. The one thing that all these disorders have in common is that they are frequently caused by allergies. What to? Well, a growing number of doctors have noticed that these conditions are more common among people who eat a junk food diet or who consume large amounts of dairy food and the suspicion is that many of those who suffer from these allergy-related problems do so because of their diet. It is now widely believed among doctors that many people whose diet includes too many refined foods, too many additive-rich foods and not enough fresh fruit or vegetables would be much healthier if they changed their eating habits.

Anaemia

The type of anaemia caused by eating a diet which contains too little iron is remarkably common in the Western world. The human body can absorb iron more easily when the iron is consumed along with a diet which is rich in vitamin C.

Anxiety

Many who suffer from constant or recurrent anxiety live on a diet which contains too little vitamin B and so if you are an anxiety sufferer you may be able to improve your resistance to anxiety by increasing your consumption of vitamin B rich foods. Anxiety sufferers should also be able to reduce their symptoms by cutting down the amount of sugar they eat and by drinking less caffeine-rich drinks.

Asthma

The incidence of asthma has trebled in the last two or three generations and it is now widely acknowledged that there are probably two main reasons for this: the pollution of our atmosphere with industrial waste chemicals and carbon monoxide gases and general poor eating habits. (There is a third reason: the fact that doctors are today much quicker to diagnose asthma, and to regard every patient who wheezes as being a full blown asthmatic.) The problem which seems most likely to be responsible for the increase in the incidence of asthma is our increased consumption of dairy products such as milk, butter and cheese (though a diet which is rich in fatty meat is also very likely to trigger off asthma attacks). Many patients who suffer from asthma have found that their symptoms improve if they change to a diet which contains more fruit, nuts and vegetables and less dairy products and meat. In an emergency, by the way, it is possible to obtain some slight relief from the wheezing associated with asthma by consuming a drink which is rich in caffeine

Anaemia

The type of anaemia caused by eating a diet which contains too little iron is remarkably common in the Western world. The human body can absorb iron more easily when the iron is consumed along with a diet which is rich in vitamin C.

Anxiety

Many who suffer from constant or recurrent anxiety live on a diet which contains too little vitamin B and so if you are an anxiety sufferer you may be able to improve your resistance to anxiety by increasing your consumption of vitamin B rich foods. Anxiety sufferers should also be able to reduce their symptoms by cutting down the amount of sugar they eat and by drinking less caffeine-rich drinks.

Asthma

The incidence of asthma has trebled in the last two or three generations and it is now widely acknowledged that there are probably two main reasons for this: the pollution of our atmosphere with industrial waste chemicals and carbon monoxide gases and general poor eating habits. (There is a third reason: the fact that doctors are today much quicker to diagnose asthma, and to regard every patient who wheezes as being a full blown asthmatic.) The problem which seems most likely to be responsible for the increase in the incidence of asthma is our increased consumption of dairy products such as milk, butter and cheese (though a diet which is rich in fatty meat is also very likely to trigger off asthma attacks). Many patients who suffer from asthma have found that their symptoms improve if they change to a diet which contains more fruit, nuts and vegetables and less dairy products and meat. In an emergency, by the way, it is possible to obtain some slight relief from the wheezing associated with asthma by consuming a drink which is rich in caffeine a powerful drug which is an effective bronchodilator. Coffee, tea and cola drinks may all provide short term emergency relief for asthma sufferers.

Atherosclerosis

Doctors around the world now agree that your chances of developing atherosclerosis — or clogged up arteries — are closely linked to what you choose to eat. If you eat too much fat (and, in particular, too much saturated animal fat) and too much sugar then your risk of developing atherosclerosis and suffering from heart disease, stroke or high blood pressure will be dramatically increased. There is also evidence to show that a high caffeine consumption can also increase your chances of suffering from atherosclerosis. You can reduce your chances of developing atherosclerosis — and the associated disorders — by increasing your consumption of high fibre foods such as oat bran and of vegetables. You may also be able to help yourself by eating more beans, garlic, onions and live yoghurt.

Cataracts

You can reduce your risk of developing a cataract by keeping your intake of sugar as low as possible.

Constipation

A diet that is rich in sugar and meat will increase your chances of suffering from constipation. You can reduce your chances of suffering from constipation by increasing the amount of roughage or fibre that you eat.

Depression

If you suffer from depression you may also be suffering from a shortage of vitamin B.

Diabetes

If you already have diabetes then you may be able to reduce your need for drug therapy by cutting down your consumption of sugar and fat rich foods. Cutting down your consumption of foods of this type may also help you not to develop diabetes. Individuals with a family history of diabetes who want to reduce their chances of suffering from the disorder should, therefore, eat less fat and less sugar rich foods. A diet which is high in fibre and complex carbohydrates is excellent. The fibre helps by slowing down the rate at which sugar is absorbed. You must, of course, see your doctor if you are a diabetic before you make any change to your diet.

Gall Bladder Disease (Including Gallstones)

The high incidence of gallstones in Western society is very closely linked to the type of food we eat. Most of us eat far too much fat and far too little fibre. We also tend to eat far too much food in general. Gallstones are an almost inevitable consequence of all this overeating and self indulgence. You can reduce your risk of developing gallstones (or suffering from any symptoms associated with their existence) by keeping your fat consumption down, reducing your consumption of refined carbohydrates, controlling your weight, increasing your intake of fibre rich foods such as fresh fruit, fresh vegetables and whole grain cereals. There is, in addition, some evidence showing that eating a regular breakfast will help to reduce your chances of suffering from gall bladder problems. Some experts also claim that food allergies can sometimes lead to gall bladder problems. The three foods most commonly blamed for allergies leading to gall bladder trouble are eggs, pork and onions. If you suffer from a gall bladder problem you should (in addition to cutting down your fat intake and increasing the amount of fibre you eat) reduce your intake of these three foods for a while to see if your symptoms disappear.

Gout

Gout can be triggered off by foods which are rich in purines so if you suffer from gout you would probably be sensible to avoid meat extracts, game, asparagus, spinach, strawberries, rhubarb, fish roe, herring, salmon, whitebait, liver, kidneys and sweetbreads. You will probably also benefit by cutting down on your consumption of protein rich foods and by limiting your intake of fish, peas and beans. Gout sufferers are also sometimes intolerant of carbonated drinks, beer, sparkling wines, port, champagne and, indeed, other types of alcohol.

Headaches

Stress, tension and anxiety are undoubtedly the commonest causes of headaches. Food is the second commonest cause although most headache sufferers only seem to get problems because of a sensitivity to specific types of food. Alcohol, chocolate, fatty foods and additive rich foods are among the most frequent causes of headaches. Many patients who suffer from food-related headaches are able to deal with their problem permanently by keeping a diary, finding out which foods seem to trigger their symptoms, and then eliminating those foods from their diet. Caffeine — usually drunk as strong coffee or as tea — is a common cause of headaches. In some cases caffeine linked headaches are caused by drinking coffee or tea. In other cases the headaches occur as withdrawal headaches — when the victim hasn't drunk any coffee or tea for a while.

Heart disease

The link between fat intake and heart disease was first officially established back in 1953. Since then a great deal more evidence has been collected to support the contention that fat intake is one of the major factors in the development of heart disease. Virtually every major, independent scientific and medical committee in the world now agrees that saturated fats cause heart disease. And just about every expert in the world agrees that we would all be wise to cut down our consumption of fat — and, in particular, of saturated fat. Despite this agreement, many people have continued to eat lots of fat and there is little doubt that this is a result of the efforts of pressure groups working for those industries trying to boost the sales of dairy products and meat.

I have no doubt at all that every year thousands of men and women around the world die prematurely — often in their thirties and forties — largely because they have been encouraged to eat fatty food.

The 'credit' for this disgraceful state of affairs must, in my view, go to the food manufacturers and their lobbyists — and to the politicians who have allowed the lobbyists to pressure them into inaction. The propaganda experts — hired by those industries which have a vested interest in ensuring that we all continue to eat lots of butter, eggs and fatty meat (washed down with full cream milk) — have funded a number of extremely effective campaigns. Sometimes attempts are made to exert pressure in other ways. For example, after I appeared on one British TV station and told viewers that a high fat diet containing too much butter and milk could lead to heart disease the station received a letter from an executive of the Butter Information Council. The writer of the letter pointed out that his organisation had been about to spend a large sum of money on TV advertising, and that this plan had 'come under review' as a result of my remarks. Cutting down your consumption of fat will cut down your calorie intake, improve your health and ensure that your heart remains in the best possible condition. Saturated fat won't just clog up your blood vessels; it will also reduce the efficiency with which your red blood cells carry oxygen around your body, and it will pick up and accumulate waste products which should be excreted. To keep your heart healthy reduce the amount of fatty meat that you eat and keep down your intake of high fat dairy products.

Heartburn

Under normal circumstances the acid mixture that helps to digest food within the stomach is kept away from the oesophagus by a sphincter which allows food to travel down into the stomach but doesn't allow food and acid to travel upwards into the gullet. The acid in the stomach is strong enough to dissolve steak (or burn holes in your carpet) and the oesophagus simply isn't made to cope with it. The sphincter is important. If the sphincter which usually divides the oesophagus from the stomach in this way doesn't do its job properly acid can sometimes splash upwards and irritate the oesophageal mucosa. The technical term for this is gastro-oesophageal reflux and the word 'heartburn' is very descriptive. The burning sensation rises up from the stomach and radiates to the upper chest — sometimes producing such a vicious pain that it can be confused with a heart attack.

Even when the sphincter is in good working condition acid can irritate the oesophagus when you lie down or bend over. Naturally enough, therefore, individuals who have a weak sphincter at that point will find that they suffer far more when they are lying flat or bending over than they do when they are standing up straight. Being overweight can increase the risk of heartburn. As can eating a diet which contains too much fat. And despite the fact that heartburn usually has a solid physical cause there are many individuals who suffer from this symptom purely as a result of stress.

As many as one in ten adults has reflux symptoms on a daily basis. Nearly half get symptoms at least once a month. Pregnant women are particularly at risk and around three quarters of pregnant women suffer from heartburn at some point in their pregnancy. Heartburn is a widespread and major problem.

There are a number of things that you can do to protect yourself from heartburn (whether you've already got it or not). Avoiding smoking is a good start. Losing excess weight helps.

Here are my top tips for dealing with heartburn:

1. Avoid coffee and tea.

2. Avoid fatty foods.

3. Avoid spicy foods.

4. Avoid chocolate.

5. Avoid peppermint.

6. Avoid drinks which are too hot or too cold.

7. Avoid alcohol.

8. Avoid fizzy drinks.

9. Eat brown rice, buckwheat and legumes.

10. Vitamins A and D are believed to help.

11. Don't lie down within three hours of eating a meal.

12. Try sleeping on an extra pillow.

13. Eat small meals.

14. Avoid unnecessary stress — and learn to deal with the unavoidable stresses in your life more effectively.

15. Antacid preparations will neutralise acid in the stomach and provide a fairly instant relief. Liquid preparations coat the oesophagus effectively. The snag is that the stomach can react by producing more acid — meaning that the relief can be short lived. The stomach is likely to respond to antacids in tablet form by producing a lower level of acidity — the desired effect may take more time but the effect should last longer.

High Blood Pressure
Up to 25% of the world's population have high blood pressure.

Only 50% of those individuals know that they suffer from high blood pressure. Only 25% are being treated. And only half ofthose are being treated effectively. But high blood pressure is a major killer — an important cause of heart disease and strokes. If you suffer from high blood pressure you may be able to control your problem simply by eating more carefully. You should eat a low fat, high fibre diet and you should reduce your intake of salt as much as you can and increase your intake of potassium. Even if you don't suffer from high blood pressure but have a family history of high blood pressure you should reduce your salt intake. You can do this by not adding salt to foods that are being cooked and by leaving the salt cellar off the table. Other flavourings which can be used instead of salt include lemon juice, parsley, garlic, horseradish and tarragon.

You should also avoid or reduce your consumption of the following foods:

* Processed foods in general
* Canned foods
* Junk food
* Crisps
* Salted peanuts
* Salted biscuits
* Salted butter
* Salted cheese
* Sausages
* Bacon

Just as there is evidence to show that too much salt has an adverse effect on some patients with high blood pressure so there is also evidence that some patients with blood pressure problems may be helped by increasing their intake of potassium.

Foods that are rich in potassium include:

* Apples
* Apricots
* Asparagus
* Bananas
* Beans
* Brussels Sprouts
* Cabbage
* Corn on the Cob
* Dates
* Grapefruit
* Oranges
* Peas
* Peppers

* Prunes

* Potatoes

* Radishes

* Raisins

For more information about high blood pressure see my book *High Blood Pressure,* published by the European Medical Journal.

Indigestion

Indigestion is one of the commonest of all diseases. The chances are that there is a sufferer in your family. Most sufferers simply head straight for the bathroom cabinet or the local chemist's shop and take a few slugs from a bottle of white medicine.

Traditional stomach remedies usually work well because they contain a substance which counteracts the powerful acid that is causing the pain. But swallowing a few gulps of white medicine after your symptoms develop only provides an immediate and short term answer and there is a real risk that if you don't do something to stop your indigestion developing you will eventually end up with a stomach ulcer.

Since what you eat — and how you eat it — is largely responsible for the pains of indigestion, here are some tips on exactly how you can reduce your chances of developing indigestion. Even if you're not already a sufferer you'll benefit by following this advice.

1. Remember that eating regular meals is better for you than going for long periods without food. If you eat regularly then the acid that accumulates in your stomach will have nothing to work on — except your stomach lining.

2. Eat slowly. Put down your knife and fork between mouthfuls — that should slow you down.

3. Put small amounts into your mouth. If you stuff huge amounts of food into your mouth then you'll swallow without chewing. Chewing is an essential part of the digestive process.

4. When you've finished a meal have a short rest. Give your stomach time to finish its job before you start chasing around again.

5. Don't read or watch TV while you're eating. If you concentrate on what you're doing when you have a meal then you'll be much more likely to know when you've had enough to eat. Overeating is a common cause of stomach problems.

6. Don't let other people push you into eating more than you want. Be prepared to leave food on the side of your plate if you've had enough.

7. Avoid any foods which upset your stomach. The sort of foods that can cause upsets are: all fried foods, fizzy drinks, alcohol, strong tea or coffee, fatty foods; spicy foods, unripe fruit, very hot or very cold foods, tough food that can't be chewed easily, pickles, sprouts, radishes, cucumber, coarse bread, biscuits or cereals, nuts and dried fruit.

8. Finally, remember that tobacco smoke will irritate your stomach too.

If you suffer from recurrent or persistent indigestion then you should, of course, see your GP. There are powerful drugs available which can be used to help treat this problem without recourse to surgery.

Infections

Your body will be better able to fight off infections if you eat a diet which contains very little fat and very little sugar but good amounts of vitamins A, B and C. There is, in addition, now some evidence to show that eating a diet which contains garlic and live yoghurt will help your body fight off infection.

Insomnia

In order to sleep better and more soundly you should avoid caffeine and cows' milk and keep your consumption of alcohol down.

Irritable Bowel Syndrome (IBS)

Some experts claim that at one time or another as many as one in three people suffer from irritable bowel syndrome. Children under ten can get it and there are many sufferers in their seventies and eighties. Irritable bowel syndrome probably affects as many people as toothache or the common cold. It is also one of the most commonly misdiagnosed of all diseases — and one of the most badly treated. Once it has developed it hardly ever disappears completely.

That's the bad news.

The good news is twofold.

First, irritable bowel syndrome isn't dangerous or life threatening; it doesn't turn into anything more serious, it won't turn into cancer and it won't kill you or even threaten your life.

The symptoms associated with irritable bowel syndrome may be exhausting, irritating, worrying and disabling but there is no underlying deadly pathology.

And second, although it does tend to hang around — once you have got it you've probably got it for life — irritable bowel syndrome can be controlled. There is no quick, simple, reliable cure because there is no clearly defined cause. But although you may not be able to conquer IBS completely — and make the symptoms disappear — you *can* control it.

The primary symptoms are the ones which involve the bowel itself and what goes on inside it. Pain is probably the most obvious of these symptoms — though it is also one of the most variable. It is often a colicky, spasmodic sort of pain which comes and goes in waves; it can affect just about any part of the abdomen and it frequently fades a little when the sufferer goes to the toilet. Bowel irregularities are common too. Most sufferers complain of diarrhoea — which can sometimes be quite sudden and explosive — but, oddly enough, constipation is also a common symptom. Sometimes the two problems alternate.

The other very common bowel problem associated with this complaint is wind and this really is typical. Most sufferers complain that their tummies swell up so much that their clothes don't fit them properly. Many complain of embarrassing rumblings and gurglings and other noises and of the social problems associated with escaping wind.

In a survey of irritable bowel syndrome sufferers which was published in the *British Medical Journal* it was found that every single patient with this problem complained of these three symptoms: abdominal pain, abdominal distension caused by wind and an abnormal bowel habit.

Next, there are the secondary symptoms which affect a lot of sufferers but which don't affect all patients. You're almost certain to have the three primary symptoms but you are unlikely to have all of these secondary symptoms.

One or two of the secondary symptoms are caused by the wind that is so widely associated with irritable bowel syndrome and these will probably come and go as the wind comes and goes. Symptoms in this category include a feeling of being full all the time and not being able to eat very much, a constant feeling of nausea, heartburn and indigestion. Back pains of one sort or another are also fairly commonplace and these too are frequently a result of wind accumulating in the intestines. It is even quite common for irritable bowel syndrome sufferers to complain of urinary frequency and other bladder problemscaused by pressure produced by wind in the intestines.

Last, but certainly not least, there are the mental symptoms. Anxiety, depression and irritability are all common, but the one mental symptom that really seems to affect irritable bowel syndrome patients more than any other is tiredness.

Even though you may be quite convinced that you are suffering from irritable bowel syndrome you shouldn't make the diagnosis by yourself without visiting your doctor. Although irritable bowel syndrome is probably the commonest of all bowel problems today there are other problems which can cause bowel symptoms and only by visiting your doctor can you be absolutely sure that you have got the diagnosis right.

Stress is one cause of irritable bowel syndrome. The other is diet.

In the last century or so the people who produce, market and sell our food have changed our diet almost beyond recognition.

173

Today most of us tend to eat a bland over-refined diet that contains very little natural roughage. And the result is that our bowels can't cope very well with this change — they haven't had time to adapt and so they struggle. Our grandparents ate a diet that contained lots of raw, natural foods. We tend to live on prepackaged, convenience foods that may be rich in vitamins and minerals but which are dangerously short on fibre.

To control your IBS properly you need to take a long, cool, careful and critical look at your diet.

You will almost certainly benefit if you gradually increase the amount of fibre that you eat. To do this start eating wholemeal bread or high bran cereals. Eat wholewheat pasta, brown rice, oats — in porridge for example — and more fresh vegetables and fruit, though if you suffer a lot from wind you will probably be wise to avoid any vegetables — such as sprouts — which seem to give you a lot of wind. Nibble fruit and nuts instead of chocolate and sweets.

Try to cut down your fat intake too. If you eat meat then cut off the visible fat. Don't add fat when cooking and grill,bake, steam, poach, casserole and boil rather than roasting or frying. Finally, you may find that you can help yourself by cutting out all dairy products — milk, butter and cheese.

For more information about IBS see my book *Relief from Irritable Bowel Syndrome* published by the European Medical Journal.

Kidney Stones

You can help reduce your risk of developing kidney stones by avoiding sugar and meat and by following a high fibre diet. You should also avoid milk and caffeine and drink plenty of fresh water.

Osteoporosis

There are probably more misconceptions about osteoporosis than about any other disease.

Myth 1: Osteoporosis is a disease which exclusively or largely affects women.

Myth 2: Osteoporosis is directly caused by, or is an inevitable consequence, of menopausal changes in circulating hormone levels.

Myth 3: Osteoporosis (and the risk of developing bone fractures) can be safely prevented and/or cured by swallowing large quantities of calcium — ideally either in the form of dairy produce or calcium tablets.

These myths are well established as apparent facts but are relatively easy to disprove. Osteoporosis is not exclusive to women and it is not caused by the menopause (or even associated with it directly). And a high intake of milk doesn't appear to help avoid bone loss, osteoporosis or fractures. A major study of 77,761 women aged between 34 and 59 showed that women who drank three or more glasses of milk a day had no fewer hip or arm fractures than those who drank little or no milk. The results also showed that fracture rates for milk drinkers were significantly higher for those women who consumed three or more glasses of milk a day.

The three myths were, of course, developed quite deliberately for very specific commercial purposes.

The truth about maintaining strong bones (and avoiding osteoporosis) is quite different to these myths.

One recent study has shown that vegetarians absorb and retain more calcium from foods than do non-vegetarians and other studies cite lower rates of osteoporosis in vegetarians than in non-vegetarians. Vegetarian and vegan diets may actually protect against osteoporosis. The wisest course is to obtain dietary calcium from a wide range of sources. Possible calcium sources include: broccoli,

175

molasses, chick peas, dried figs, tofu, endive, cabbage, kale, spinach and many different types of beans (including soya beans and vegetarian baked beans).

Probably the simplest way to make sure you get plenty of calcium is to eat plenty of dark green leafy vegetables.

Many factors in addition to, and other than, the consumption of calcium play a significant part in the development and maintenance of healthy bones. These factors have not been widely discussed or promoted in recent years and I find it difficult to avoid the conclusion that this has been because these other factors have not been promoted by individuals working for or on behalf of commercial organisations. Put quite simply, it is easy to make money out of selling calcium (either in the form of milk or calcium tablets) but not easy to make money out of offering good advice which does not involve the sale of a product.

It is, for example, vital to remember that there are, in addition to calcium, around twenty other essential nutrients — including a variety of vitamins and minerals — which are required before the body can build and maintain healthy bones. If the diet is deficient in any of these nutrients then the bones will become weak. You don't need to take supplements to obtain these essential nutrients: all you need is a good, balanced diet that includes plenty of fruit and vegetables (preferably organically grown and genetically unmodified).

It is also important to remember that apart from ensuring a reasonable intake of calcium (best done without dairy produce) it is also necessary to reduce the loss of calcium from your body.

There are a number of things you can do to minimise calcium loss.

First, you should avoid tobacco (smokers have a hip fracture risk 40% higher than non smokers).

Second, don't drink more than two cups of coffee or tea a day and keep your intake of alcohol down.

Third, you should be aware that a sedentary lifestyle may lead to calcium losses so take regular, gentle exercise which you enjoy. Exercising just three times a week will help to strengthen bone density noticeably. The best forms of exercise for strengthening the bones include weight training and walking uphill or cycling uphill. (Remember that you should not exercise if it is painful and you should always consult your doctor before starting an exercise programme or altering your exercise habits.)

Fourth you should keep your intake of salt down.

Fifth, it is important to avoid constant dieting. The evidence shows that whenever someone diets and loses weight he or she will also lose bone. Since women tend to diet more than men this is a problem which affects women more than men. Clearly, therefore, women who have spent much of their lives dieting, regaining weight and dieting again will have lost a good deal of bone by the time they reach the menopause. (And the arrival of the menopause will be a mere coincidence.)

It is also important to be aware that the human body also needs vitamin D to make healthy bones. Obtaining vitamin D is easy: ten or twenty minutes of sun on face, hands and arms, taken just three times a week, should produce all the vitamin D the body needs. People with dark skin, or those who live in cloudy or smoggy areas or in northern areas may need slightly more exposure.

Finally, and most importantly, you should be aware that eating animal protein results in withdrawal of calcium from the bones into the bloodstream. The calcium is then excreted in the urine and lost.

Eating large amounts of animal protein can dramatically increase the rate at which the body loses calcium. This is probably the most important single secret in the battle against osteoporosis and bone fractures. It is a secret which has been deliberately suppressed and hidden by those industries which have a vested interest in selling their 'solutions' to this problem — and by the meat industry which is, not surprisingly, nervous about the long term consequences to its own profitability once the secret becomes widely known.

The truth is that meat consumption is one of the most important factors in the development of bone loss, osteoporosis and fractures.

(Incidentally, meat protein is a very poor source of calcium. Strawberries contain more calcium than rump steak or corned beef.)

A report which was published in the *American Journal of Clinical Nutrition* in 1994 showed that when volunteers switch from a typical Western diet to one which does not include animal protein calcium losses are halved. A study of the health of 85,900 women aged between 35 and 59 showed that an increase in consumption of animal protein was associated with an increased risk of forearm fracture. No such association was found for the consumption of vegetable protein. Women who consume five or more servings of red meat each week have a significantly increased risk of forearm fracture when compared with women who eat red meat less than once a week.

Moreover, there is strong evidence to suggest that in those countries where calcium consumption is low and bone fracture rates are also low the key factor may well be the level of animal protein consumption.

For example, according to an article in *The Vegan* magazine (published by the Vegan Society in Britain) hip fracture rates in Beijing (China) are among the lowest in the world de-spite the fact that the mean daily intake of calcium in China is only 540 mg per person per day. (In the US the comparable figure is 1140 mg.) The big nutritional difference between the two countries lies in the amount of animal protein which is consumed. A staggering 70% of the protein consumed in the US is from animals. In China just 7% of the protein consumed is from animals.

In addition to all this it is important to remember that environmental toxins and mental stresses can also interfere with the body's ability to function effectively — and, therefore, its ability to build new bone. And the surgical removal of the ovaries can have a damaging effect on the body's bone building ability.

Osteoporosis is a nasty disease. But it is a disease largely created and sustained by our way of life. As with so many other disorders our slick 'in a bottle', modern solutions often simply add additional problems to existing ones. In my view the best way to avoid osteoporosis — and to deal with it — is to be aware of the real causes and to do something about them.

I believe that osteoporosis is yet another twentieth century lifestyle disease which can, not surprisingly perhaps, best be avoided (and conquered) through a change in lifestyle.

Premenstrual Syndrome
Women who suffer from painful, uncomfortable or unpleasant symptoms just before a period may be able to help themselves by reducing their intake of caffeine, milk, salt and sugar.

Restless Legs Syndrome
Many women complain that while they lie in bed at night their legs twitch. This is called the 'restless legs syndrome'. It is one of the oldest of all disorders and was first described over 300 years ago. Caffeine is believed to be one of the major causes today. To avoid

the problem try drinking less — or weaker — coffee or tea. If you spend much of your time sitting down then mild exercise will probably help.

Rheumatoid Arthritis

There is evidence now available to show that sufferers from rheumatoid arthritis can help themselves by avoiding meat and following a vegetarian diet. You may also benefit from limiting the amount of fresh fruit that you eat.

For more information on arthritis see my book *How To Conquer Arthritis* published by the European Medical Journal.

Strokes

If you want to cut down your risk of having a stroke you should eat more fresh vegetables, more fibre rich cereals and more fresh fruit and avoid foods which are rich in fat — particularly saturated fat. In practice this means avoiding red meat and dairy products.

Tinnitus

It is sometimes possible to ease this exceptionally annoying problem of noises in the ears by cutting down your consumption of fat and sugar.

Tooth Decay and Gum Disease

Half of all five year old children in the West have some tooth decay. Campaigns organised by governments, doctors and dentists have been successfully overshadowed by advertising campaigns run by food companies encouraging children to eat more sweets and chocolates.

The constant consumption of sugar-rich foods feeds the bacteria which produce the acid which attacks teeth and starts the process of decay. By eating fewer sugar-rich foods and by increasing your consumption of fresh fruit and vegetables you will be able dramatically to reduce the risk of suffering from either tooth decay or gum disease.

Ulcers (gastric and duodenal)
cf Indigestion

Varicose Veins
You are more likely to develop and suffer from varicose veins if you eat a high fat, low fibre diet. Constipation and obesity — both problems which are associated with a high fat, low fibre diet — dramatically increase the risk of varicose veins developing.

Wind
This problem is one of the commonest of all health problems — affecting well over half of the population. Doctors really don t understand much about, it. And can't do much to deal with it.

The normal gastrointestinal tract is said to contain between 100 and 200 millilitres of gas under normal circumstances. During an ordinary sort of day a normal individual will often produce 1 to 2 litres of gas. It is, therefore, quite obvious that there must be a tendency for wind to pass out of the gastrointestinal tract at one end or the other. (Wind consists of 250 different gases. The study of flatulence is called flatology. The most astonishing fact about wind is that it is normal to 'break wind' at around 100 mph.)

Wind is produced within the gastrointestinal tract as food is digested, and some foods are more likely than others to result in the production of large quantities of wind. Brussels sprouts and cabbage are fairly widely recognised as offending vegetables and beans, of course, have a tremendous reputation in this respect.

It is, however, important to understand that not all of the wind in the gastrointestinal tract is a result of the normal digestive process.

Some of the wind that causes such embarrassing noises gets into the intestinal tract in the same way that food gets in: it is swallowed. People who chew gum, smoke cigarettes or eat too quickly will often swallow air as will those individuals who gulp in air as a nervous habit. Indeed, two thirds of the gas in your body is probably swallowed air. You're likely to swallow too much air if you gulp hot drinks or sip drinks through a straw. Habits like sucking mints can also cause wind to accumulate. Fizzy drinks are an obvious cause of wind. Chewing with an open mouth or talking with your mouth full increases the likelihood of wind too. Foods that are likely to cause wind include: beans, broccoli, cabbage, raisins, bananas, popcorn, peanuts, onions, chocolate, coffee and milk.

Things Every Wind Sufferer Should Know

1. Swallowing air is a common (and unconscious) cause of bloating.

2. Bacterial metabolism of food in the intestine may cause gas. Some foods — e.g. beans and cabbage — are worse than others.

3. Eating simple sugars may make wind worse. Foods to avoid in particular include table sugar, sweets, biscuits, cakes, crisps, white bread and processed breakfast cereals. Remember that around 80% of the sugar we eat annually comes from packaged foods.

4. Tolerance to the amount of gas in the intestine varies enormously. Some people are particularly sensitive to it.

5. Eating too quickly can result in air being swallowed and chewing gum and smoking cigarettes can also both result in more air being swallowed.

6. Wind sufferers should avoid the following foods: milk and dairy produce, fresh fruits, some vegetables. Carbonated beverages may make things worse — as may antacids such as baking soda.

7. Some people benefit by eating more fibre. Others benefit by eating less.

8. If the gas coming out smells unpleasant then you are probably eating too much animal protein (or failing to digest it properly). Animal proteins contain large amounts of sulphur — which smells a lot.

9. Too much fat encourages inflammation in the intestinal tract. And this can cause bloating.

10. The foods we are most likely to be sensitive to (and which are most likely to cause problems) are the foods to which we are addicted. So, if you can't stop eating chocolate you are probably sensitive to it. If cheese is your favourite food then you may well be sensitive to dairy produce.

11. Lactose intolerance affects around 1 in 7 individuals of Northern or Middle European descent — and up to 95% of those of African, American, Asian origin.

12. Drinking water can help reduce bloating. You need two to three litres a day. Coffee, tea and cola drinks don't count because they may make things worse.

CHAPTER FOURTEEN

TWENTY ONE REASONS FOR BEING A VEGETARIAN

Vegetarianism is the fastest growing trend in the developed world.

Here are 21 reasons why you should think about turning vegetarian too.

1. Avoiding meat is one of the best and simplest ways to cut down your fat consumption. Modern farm animals are deliberately fattened up to increase profits. Eating fatty meat increases your chances of having a heart attack or developing cancer.

2. Every minute of every working day thousands of animals are killed in slaughterhouses. Many animals are bled to death. Pain and misery are commonplace. In America alone 500,000 animals are killed for meat every hour.

3. There are millions of cases of food poisoning recorded every year. The vast majority of all those cases are caused by eating meat.

4. Meat contains absolutely nothing — no proteins, vitamins or minerals — that the human body cannot obtain perfectly happily from a vegetarian diet.

5. African countries — where millions are starving to death — export grain to the developed world so that animals can be fattened for the dining tables of the affluent nations.

6. 'Meat' can include the tail, head, feet, rectum and spinal cord of an animal.

7. A sausage may contain ground-up intestines. How can anyone be sure that the intestines are empty when they are ground up? Do you really want to eat the content of a pig's intestines?

8. If we eat the plants we grow — instead of feeding them to animals — the world's food shortage will disappear virtually overnight. One hundred acres of land will produce enough beef for 20 people but enough wheat to feed 240 people.

9. Every day tens of millions of one day old male chicks are killed because they will not be able to lay eggs. There are no rules about how this mass slaughter takes place. Some are crushed or suffocated to death. Many are used for fertiliser or fed to other animals.

10. Animals who die for your dinner table die alone, in terror, in sadness and in pain. The killing is merciless and inhumane.

11. It is much easier to become — and stay — slim if you are vegetarian. (By 'slim' I do not mean 'abnormally slender' or 'underweight' but, rather, an absence of excess weight.)

12. Half the rainforests in the world have been destroyed to clear ground to graze cattle to make beefburgers. The burning of the forests contributes 20% of all greenhouse gases. Roughly 1,000 species a year become extinct because of the destruction of the rain forests. Approximately 260 million acres of US forest have been cleared to grow crops to feed cattle so that people can eat meat.

13. Every year 440 million tons of grain are fed to livestock — so that the world's rich can eat meat. At the same time 500 million people in poor countries are starving to death. Every six seconds someone in the world starves to death because people in the west are eating meat. Approximately 60 million people a year die of starvation. All those lives could be saved — because those people could eat the grain used to fatten cattle and other farm animals — if Americans ate 10% less meat.

14. The world's fresh water shortage is being made worse by animal farming. And meat producers are the biggest polluters of water. It takes 2,500 gallons of water to produce one pound of meat. If the meat industry in America wasn't supported by the taxpayer paying a large proportion of its water costs then hamburger meat would cost $35 a pound.

15. If you eat meat you are consuming hormones that were fed to the animals. No one knows what effect those hormones will have on your health. In some parts of the world as many as one in four hamburgers contain growth hormones that were originally given to cattle.

16. The following diseases are commoner among meat eaters: anaemia, appendicitis, arthritis, breast cancer, cancer of the colon, cancer of the prostate, constipation, diabetes, gallstones, gout, high blood pressure, indigestion, obesity, piles, strokes and varicose veins. Lifelong vegetarians visit hospital 22% less often than meat eaters — and for shorter stays. Vegetarians have a 20% lower blood

cholesterol levels than meat eaters — and this reduces heart attack and cancer risks considerably.

17. Some farmers use tranquillisers to keep animals calm. Others routinely use antibiotics to stave off infection. When you eat meat you are eating those drugs. Considerably more than half of all the antibiotics sold are given by farmers to healthy animals and the percentage of staphylococci infections resistant to penicillin went up from 13% in 1960 to 91% in 1988.

18. In a lifetime the average meat eater will consume 36 pigs, 36 sheep and 750 chickens and turkeys. Do you want that much carnage on your conscience?

19. Animals suffer from pain and fear just as much as you do. How would you like to spend your last hours locked in a truck, packed into a cage with hundreds of other terrified animals and then cruelly pushed into a blood soaked death chamber. Anyone who eats meat condones and supports the way animals are treated.

20. Animals which are a year old are often far more rational — and capable of logical thought — than six week old babies. Pigs and sheep are far more intelligent than small children. Eating dead animals is barbaric.

21. Vegetarians are fitter than meat eaters. Many of the world's most successful athletes are vegetarian.

What can I eat?

Many people are put off becoming vegetarian because they can't think what they will be able to eat if they don't eat meat.

A quick trip to your local supermarket will, however, show that there are not only many different fruits and vegetables available but that because vegetarianism is growing rapidly there are many ready-made vegetarian meals on sale.

You will also find many 'meat substitute' meals available. You can buy vegetarian sausages and hamburgers, and stews and curries made with soya have a similar texture to meals made with meat.

Vegetarian Recipes

Here are some simple, meat free recipes designed to show you that life without meat need not be dull.

SPAGHETTI NAPOLETANA

Serves 2

3oz/90g wholemeal spaghetti

1 tablespoon oil

2oz/60g mushrooms, chopped

1/2 green pepper, chopped

1 small carrot, chopped

1 small clove garlic, chopped

1 small onion, chopped

4oz/250g tinned tomatoes

1 tablespoon tomato puree

herbs and seasoning to taste

Cook the spaghetti in boiling water. Fry the vegetables in oil for 5 minutes. Add the tomatoes, the tomato puree and herbs and seasoning to taste. Cook for a few more minutes. Drain the spaghetti and serve with the thick vegetable sauce poured over it.

PARISIAN SALAD

Serves 2

1 orange, peeled and segmented
1 carrot, grated
1/2oz/15g almonds, chopped
2oz/60g celery, chopped
1 stick French bread

Break the orange segments in half, then mix the first four ingredients together. Eat with the French bread stick.

SAVOURY DUTCH CAKES

Serves 2

8oz/250g potatoes, cooked in their skins
nutmeg to taste
ground black pepper to taste
1 tablespoon soya milk
1 medium onion, finely chopped
4oz/125g cooked green vegetables

If you intend to use the oven, preheat to 180 C (350 F/gas mark 4) and grease a baking tray. Peel the potatoes, then mash with the nutmeg and black pepper. Add the soya milk. Fry the onion without oil in a non-stick pan until tender. Mix together the potatoes, green vegetables and onion and form them into four round cakes. Bake for 10 minutes or grill under a moderate heat for 15 minutes.

GOLDEN VEGETABLE PARCELS

Serves 2

1/4 pint/150ml soya milk

1/2 tablespoon cornflour

1/2 tablespoon chopped parsley

black pepper to taste

selection of leftover cooked vegetables

4oz/125g shortcrust puff pastry

Preheat the oven to 220 C (425 F/gas mark 7) and grease a baking tray. Mix the cornflour with a little cold soya milk to make a smooth paste. Pour remaining milk into a saucepan, then add cornflour paste and heat slowly, and stir. Keep the milk on the heat until it has thickened, then add the parsley and season with black pepper. Add the cooked vegetables. Roll out the pastry on a floured surface and cut it into four squares. Put the vegetables into the centres of two of the pastry squares. Brush the edges of the squares with water, and then put the remaining squares on top to make 'parcels'. Pinch the edges together well to seal them. Transfer the parcels to the baking tray and bake for 25 minutes.

FRENCH BROCCOLI

Serves 2

1 tablespoon vegetable oil

2 spring onions, chopped

1 clove garlic crushed

1/2 teaspoon oregano

1/2 teaspoon tarragon

1 tablespoon freshly chopped parsley

pinch cayenne pepper

ground black pepper to taste

12oz/350g cooked broccoli

2oz/60g breadcrumbs

Heat the oil and sauté the onions and garlic. Add the herbs and seasonings and then the broccoli. Put the mixture into a fireproof casserole. Place the breadcrumbs on top. Grill until the top appears well browned.

HOT DEVILLED EGGS

Serves 2

2 hard-boiled eggs
1 tablespoon soya yoghurt
ground black pepper to taste
pinch of dry mustard powder
paprika to taste

Shell the eggs and cut in half lengthways. Carefully remove the yolks with a sharp knife and put to one side for use in another dish, or as a sandwich filling. Add the pepper and mustard to the yoghurt and mix until smooth. Spoon the mixture into egg white hollows and sprinkle lightly with paprika.

MILANESE PEPPERS

Serves 2

1 large red or green pepper
1 tablespoon vegetable oil 1 large onion, chopped
1 clove garlic, crushed
2 tablespoons red wine
1 tablespoon tomato puree
1 tablespoon mixed chopped rosemary, oregano, parsley and mint
4 tablespoons vegetable stock
4oz/125g pasta shapes, uncooked

1 1/2 oz/40g breadcrumbs

1 egg white

Preheat the oven to 180 C (350 F/gas mark 4) and grease a baking dish. Boil the pepper in water for 1 minute. Then cool it under running water, halve and remove the seeds. Heat the oil and sauté the onion and garlic. Add the wine, tomato puree, herbs and stock. Simmer for 10 minutes. Place the pasta shapes in a large bowl. Add the breadcrumbs and egg white, mix well, then add the cooked onion and herbs. Spoon the mixture into the pepper halves and place on a baking dish. Put the entire baking dish into a shallow tray containing a little water. Cover, and bake for 35 minutes.

OAT BRAN MUFFINS

Makes about 12 American-style muffins (small cakes, not muffins for toasting)

12oz/350g oat bran

1/2 oz/40g mixed dried fruit

(raisins, sultanas, currants, chopped dates, etc.)

1 tablespoon baking powder

1 1/2 oz/40g chopped, mixed nuts

2oz/60g sugar or equivalent artificial sweetener

8 fl. oz/250ml soya milk

2 tablespoons vegetable oil

2 egg whites

Preheat the oven to 220 C (425 F/ gas mark 7) and grease a 12-hole deep patty tin. Mix the oat bran, dried fruit, baking powder and nuts, then add the sugar. Mix the milk, oil and egg whites together and add to the oat bran mixture. Mix thoroughly and spoon the mixture evenly into the patty tins. Bake for 15-20 minutes or until the muffins are firm to press.

NUT BISCUITS

Makes about 10 biscuits

rice paper

2 egg whites

4oz/125g ground mixed nuts

30z/90g sugar

2 tablespoons ground brown rice

Preheat the oven to 180 C (350 F/gas mark 4). Grease a baking tray and line it with rice paper. Whisk the egg whites until stiff. Add the nuts, sugar and rice. Space out dollops of the mixture on the rice paper, and cook for 20-25 minutes. Serve the biscuits each with their square of rice paper.

VEGETABLE HOTPOT

Serves 2

1 tablespoon vegetable oil

1 medium onion, chopped

1 small turnip, sliced

1 large carrot, sliced

1 medium potato, sliced

4 sprouts, sliced

1 pint/600ml water

1 tablespoon soya sauce

1 tablespoon chopped fresh parsley

In a heavy saucepan fry the onion in the oil. Add the rest of the vegetables and half the water. Bring to the boil, then simmer covered for 20 minutes. Add the remaining water and the soya sauce. Just before serving add the parsley.

ROYAL SALAD

Serves 2

1 cos lettuce

2 carrots

2 tomatoes

4 radishes

2oz/60g mushrooms

4 spring onions

1/2 small green pepper

1 apple

2 tablespoons vegetable oil

1 tablespoon cider vinegar

2oz/60g walnut piece

1 oz/30g roasted peanuts

1 oz/30g raisins

Shred the lettuce. Grate and chop the vegetables and slice the apple. Combine the oil and vinegar to make a dressing and mix well with the salad. Finally, add the nuts and raisins.

WELSH MUSHROOMS

Serves 2

1/2 onion, finely chopped

1 clove garlic, finely chopped

1 tablespoon vegetable oil

8oz/250g mushrooms, chopped

dash of soya sauce

2 slices wholemeal toast

Sautéthe onion and garlic in the oil. Add the mushrooms to the pan and cook gently. Stir in the soya sauce. Serve on hot toast.

SPAGHETTI VERONA

Serves 2
oil for frying
1 onion, chopped
1 stick celery, chopped
2 tablespoons red wine
2oz/390g tin tomatoes
1 tablespoon tomato puree
1 teaspoon dried mixed Italian herbs
1/4 pint/150ml vegetable stock
6oz/175g wholewheat spaghetti

Heat the oil in a frying pan and add the onion and the celery. Add the wine and bring to the boil. Simmer for a few minutes and add the tomatoes, tomato puree and seasoning. Pour in the stock and simmer for 30 minutes. Cook the spaghetti according to the instructions on the packet, and serve immediately with the hot sauce poured over it.

PORTUGUESE HOTPOT

Serves 2
1 large potato
1 turnip
1 carrot
1 parsnip
1 onion
4oz/125g French beans

1 clove garlic

1/4 pint/ 150ml vegetable stock

1 teaspoon lemon juice

4 tomatoes, quartered

Coarsely chop all the vegetables (except the tomatoes) and steam them. Add the vegetable stock and lemon juice. Mix well and continue to cook over a low heat. When the vegetables are just about ready, add the chopped tomatoes. Cook until vegetables ready and tomatoes warmed through.

RUSSIAN CHILLI

Serves 2

1 /2 large onion, chopped

1 tablespoon vegetable oil

4oz/125g burghul (or bulgur) wheat

1 large tin tomatoes

1 tablespoon tomato puree

1 teaspoon chilli powder

ground black pepper to taste

1/2 large tin red kidney beans or 1 small tin

Saute the onion in the oil. Add the remaining ingredients except the kidney beans and simmer until the wheat is cooked but still firm. Heat the kidney beans separately and then add.

PILOT'S PIE

Serves 2

1 tablespoon vegetable oil

3oz/90g onion, chopped

3oz/90g carrot, grated

1/2 teaspoon dried thyme

1/2 tablespoon wholemeal flour

1/2 teaspoon yeast extract

4oz/125g shortcrust pastry

Preheat the oven to 190 C (375 F/gas mark 5) and grease a baking dish. Heat the oil and sauté the onion, then add the carrot and thyme and cook gently for 10 minutes. Stir in the flour and yeast extract. Leave to cool. Roll out the pastry and linethe dish with half the pastry and pile the filling into the centre. Put the remaining pastry on top and seal the edges. Make two or three small slits in the top of the pie and bake for 30 minutes.

GREEK TOMATOES

Serves 2

1 courgette

1 small aubergine

1 tablespoon vegetable oil

1 medium onion, chopped

1 clove garlic, finely chopped

1 small pepper, seeded and chopped

12oz/390g tin tomatoes

black pepper to taste

Slice the courgette and the aubergine. Leave to drain for 30 minutes. Rinse and squeeze out any excess moisture. Heat the oil in a frying pan and fry the onion and garlic. Then add all the vegetables except the tomatoes and sauté for a few minutes. Add the tomatoes and season with black pepper. Cover and simmer for 30 minutes.

WINTER SOUP

Serves 2

1 large carrot

1 large onion

2 sticks celery

half small turnip

2 medium sized potatoes

half pint/300ml vegetable stock

6 sprigs parsley

grated nutmeg and grated black pepper to taste

Chop all the vegetables and put them into a large saucepan. Add the stock and simmer for 1 hour. Just before the end of thecooking time add the parsley. Season with grated nutmeg and black pepper.

JAMAICAN RICE

Serves 2

1 tablespoon vegetable oil

half large onion, sliced

half red apple, sliced

pinch of curry powder

half pint/300ml water

4oz/125g brown rice

1 teaspoon black treacle

1 small banana, sliced

1 tablespoon desiccated coconut

Heat the oil and saute the onion and apple. Add the curry powder and water. Bring to the boil. Add the rice and treacle and cook until the water is absorbed and the rice is tender. Drain and add the banana. Sprinkle the coconut on top and heat through for a moment and then serve.

BANANA SPECIAL

Serves 2
2 bananas
1 small orange, juiced
1 oz/30g sugar
1 oz/15g polyunsaturated low fat spread

Preheat the oven to 180 C (350 F/gas mark 4), and grease an ovenproof dish. Peel the bananas, cut them in half lengthways and place them in the dish. Pour the orange juice over the bananas and sprinkle the sugar on top. Place the low fat spread on top of the bananas and cook for 15 minutes.

SPICY RED PEAR

Serves 1
1 large pear
4 tablespoons red wine
ground or whole spices — ginger, cinnamon and cloves

Peel the pear, leaving it whole with the stalk on.
Simmer in the red wine with the spices until cooked.
Serve hot.

FRUIT PUNCH
Makes about 1 pint/600ml
1 pint/600ml natural (unsweetened) pineapple juice
1 banana, sliced
1apple, chopped

1 oz/30g sesame seeds
1 oz/30g sunflower seeds
1 oz/30g raisins
1 oz/30g currants

Put all the ingredients in blender and liquidise. Keep in the refrigerator and serve chilled.

CHAPTER FIFTEEN

HEALTHY EATING — STEP ONE: EAT MORE FIBRE

Why you should increase the amount of fibre you eat

Modern food manufacturing processes make life much easier for us in many ways. Most of us don't have to grow our own food. We don't have to get up early in the morning, go out into the fields and break our backs picking the food we need to eat. We don't even have to wash our food or prepare it for cooking. We can walk into a supermarket and buy our food in boxes and tins. The preservatives used by food manufacturers mean that we can keep stocks of food on our pantry shelves so that we only have to visit the shops once a month. Life has never been easier and the big food companies spend a lot of time and energy trying to make things easier and easier for us.

Unfortunately, our bodies have failed to develop and change as fast as the food industry has changed the sort of food we eat. One major problem is that although food manufacturers have got into the habit of removing most of the roughage — which they see as waste — from our food our bodies still need that roughage in order to function properly.

When they first started doing this the food manufacturers probably thought that they were doing us a favour. After all, fibre doesn't contain any obvious nutrients. Indeed, most of the fibre we eat goes straight through our intestinal tracts and comes out — almost unchanged — at the other end. Fibre doesn't help you to build muscles and it doesn't provide essential in-gredients. However, despite this, fibre is an essential part of your daily diet; it helps to stimulate the digestive system, helps to keep food moving and gives the bowels something to squeeze. Since fibre is filling but low calorie the consumption of a diet which contains a good quantity of fibre means that you will be less likely to put on weight.

This slimming quality of fibre is enhanced by the fact that fibre slows down the absorption of sugar and helps to reduce the amount of fat that your body absorbs. Fibre may not contain any essential nutrients but it is a vital part of your diet — particularly if you want to lose excess weight and stay slim. If your diet contains too little fibre then the result will be that in addition to being overweight you may well be susceptible to a wide range of disorders as varied as cancer, diverticular disease of the bowel, appendicitis, gall stones and varicose veins.

By now it should be clear to you that the chances are high that you need to eat more fibre. If your present diet is 'average' and depends heavily on prepackaged, modern 'convenience' foods then you probably need to double your consumption of fibre. You can get all the extra fibre you need simply by taking special care about the diet you eat. You do not need to buy special fibre supplements. In fact your body will be healthier if you get the fibre it needs simply by making some fundamental alterations to the sort of things that you eat on a regular basis.

Seven ways in which increasing your fibre intake will improve your health

1. Foods which contain a large amount of fibre tend to need a lot of chewing. This will help your digestion.

2. By eating regular amounts of fibre you will help to ensure that your body gets rid of waste products more easily. A diet which

contains too little fibre is likely to lead to constipation. A diet which contains decent quantities of fibre is likely to produce healthy and regular bowel movements.

3. If you ensure that your diet contains good quantities of fibre you will reduce your chances of suffering from a wide range of digestive troubles — including appendicitis, gall stones and many bowel and stomach problems (including cancer).

4. Because foods which contain large quantities of fibre are filling (but inevitably contain relatively few calories) a diet which includes fibre-rich foods will result in you feeling full sooner and, therefore, eating less. An important advantage of this type of diet is that you will be less likely to put on excess weight and more likely to stay slim when you have become slim.

5. A diet which contains decent quantities of fibre will protect you from a variety of non-bowel disorders — including diabetes and varicose veins.

6. The fibre in the food you eat helps to reduce the amount of fat that your body absorbs. Inevitably, therefore, this means that a high fibre diet will help reduce the amount of damage which fat does to your body. By eating plenty of fibre rich foods you will reduce your chances of developing heart dis-ease, high blood pressure or a stroke.

7. Because fibre helps to absorb unwanted toxins and poisons — which you may swallow with the food you eat — a high fibre diet

will help to stop these toxic substances being absorbed into your body and making you ill.

Ten natural, healthy, easy ways to increase the amount of fibre you eat

Warning: If your fibre intake is low you should increase the amount of fibre you eat fairly gradually and slowly. If you suddenly and dramatically increase your fibre intake you may suffer from wind, pain and other signs of abdominal discomfort.

1. Try to eat more bread. Your intake of fibre will be kept highest if you eat wholemeal bread rather than white bread.

2. Eat more pasta. Again your intake of fibre will be maximised if you eat wholewheat pasta rather than white pasta.

3. Make an effort to eat more fresh, organic vegetables — a simple move which will dramatically increase your fibre intake. Try not to peel vegetables before you cook them — and certainly don't peel them too thickly. Don't cook your vegetables for too long, and cook them in as little water as possible. When preparing salads add grated raw vegetables.

4. You should also increase your intake of fresh fruit. Most fruits are rich in fibre.

5. Eat more rice. If possible eat brown rather than white rice.

6. Use wholemeal or wholewheat flour whenever possible.

7. Oats are an excellent source of fibre. You can eat them in cereals or in porridge or you can use them to make biscuits and crumbles.

8. Instead of nibbling sugar-rich sweets or fat-rich chocolates eat fibre-rich dried fruits between meals when you want a snack.

9. Try to eat more pulses (such as beans). These contain quite a lot of fibre.

10. If you must buy biscuits (which tend to contain large quantities of sugar) try to buy wholemeal biscuits — which are likely to contain more fibre.

CHAPTER SIXTEEN

HEALTHY EATING — STEP TWO: EAT LESS SUGAR

Why you should eat less sugar

Sugar has a vastly over-rated reputation as a foodstuff. Whenever small villages get cut off by snow or floods sugar is usually one of the allegedly 'staple' ingredients airlifted in by relief organisations. But sugar is a pretty useless food. It is rich in calories and will give you a quick fix if you are feeling hungry. But apart from energy you won't get much else from sugar. It is true that some types of sugar — for example blackstrap molasses — contain a few vitamins and minerals. But these ingredients aren't present in any appreciable quantities, and apart from honey (which is an exception) there isn't very much nutritional advantage to be gained by eating these types of sugar to the refined white or brown varieties which are most commonly sold. By and large sugar is sugar and most of us eat far too much of it.

It is important to realise that you won't necessarily cut down your intake of sugar simply by avoiding sweets, by not putting sugar in your tea or coffee and by using less sugar in cooking.

It is customary these days for many food manufacturers to use sugar in a whole host of unlikely ways. For example, sugar is likely to be added to tinned soup (allegedly to 'bring out the flavour' and to 'improve the texture' though you have to wonder at the quality of the soup which needs such artificial help); to tomato sauce (to make it 'smoother', though I'm not sure who decided that 'smooth' sauce was inevitably better than 'unsmoothed' sauce); to biscuits (apparently to make them 'crumblier' and 'crunchier', though I don't know about you but I don't particularly want my biscuits to crumble all over the place) and even to tinned meat to make it 'soft' (though I can't imagine anyone interested in healthy eating being prepared even to contemplate buying tinned meat).

The ubiquitous nature of sugar in refined and prepackaged foods and its image as a useful, even essential, foodstuff (and the image of it as being a rather harmless substance) means that on average we eat around 100 lbs (45kg) of sugar every year. There is no doubt that many people eat their own weight in sugar every twelve months!

Despite its image, however, sugar can be — and often is — extremely bad for you. The consumption of too much sugar frequently leads to obesity and all the problems associated with overweight. Sugar causes tooth decay and is now strongly asso-ciated with cancers of the breast and intestine.

Two ways in which eating less sugar will improve your health

1. Eating less sugar will mean that you suffer less tooth decay.

2. Keeping your sugar intake down will help you to control your weight. There is no doubt that a high sugar intake results in obesity and an increased risk of heart disease, cancer and other potentially lethal conditions.

Twelve easy ways to eat less sugar

1. Eat more natural foods — and fewer prepackaged foods. Some foods (such as fruit) do contain natural sugars but these will be mixed with lots of fibre and will be far less likely to do you harm. If you buy tinned fruits try to select the products which are packed in their own juices rather than in a sugar rich syrup.

2. Make an effort to reduce the amount of sugar you use in drinks such as tea or coffee. If you can't cope with hot drinks unless they are sweetened try using one of the many, available artificial sweeteners. As an alternative try reducing the number of cups of tea or coffee that you drink or change to other types of hot drink (for example: tea with lemon or peppermint tea which does not need sweetening).

3. Don't buy sugar rich soft drinks. Instead choose low calorie drinks or mineral water.

4. To make sure that your baby doesn't develop a 'sweet tooth' don't add sugar to milk when preparing a feed and don't buy baby foods which contain added sugar.

5. When buying fruit juices look for the natural variety rather than the ones which have added, extra sugar.

6. Buy jams and marmalades which contain less sugar than usual and when baking experiment by using slightly less sugar than recipes recommend.

7. When cooking try using spices or fruits to sweeten foods — instead of adding an enormous amount of sugar.

8. Instead of buying sweets and chocolates to nibble in between meals or during the evening choose dried fruits and nuts instead.

9. When buying biscuits choose wholemeal ones which contain relatively little sugar and eschew biscuits which are filled with cream or covered with chocolate.

10 Don't buy sweetened yoghurts. Instead buy natural, unsweetened yoghurt and to add taste and flavour add your own fruit.

11. If you are spreading jam or marmalade on bread do it thinly to reduce your sugar intake.

12. Choose fresh fruit or another alternative instead of a sugar rich pudding which is probably also rich in fat. (Remember this when eating out.)

CHAPTER SEVENTEEN

HEALTHY EATING — STEP THREE: EAT LESS FAT

Why you should eat less fat

If you eat too much cholesterol there is a risk that your body's white cells — crucial warriors in your body's immune system defences — may be damaged. And if you have lots of fat in your blood that will also affect your body's ability to deal with infections.

In a normal, healthy body white cells constantly patrol your blood stream hunting out bacteria (and stray cancer cells). If your blood stream is clogged with fat your white cells simply cannot move around effectively.

Imagine how difficult it would be for a group of lifeguards to swim through an oilslick and you'll have an idea of just how difficult it is for white cells to move through fat-soaked blood.

Incidentally, all fats are bad for your immune system but animal fats are probably worse than others, and can probably do more damage to your immune system. One of the reasons for this is the fact that animal fat is often contaminated with chemical residues — toxic and possibly carcinogenic residues of drugs consumed (accidentally or deliberately) by feeding animals.

Governments often recommend that a healthy diet should contain no more than 30% fat. I think that figure is far too high (probably because a relatively high fat diet helps keep the food industry rich and happy).

I believe that you should aim to have no more than 15-20% fat in your diet. If for some reason you need to follow a low fat diet you may wish to cut your consumption of fat to 10-15%.

Cutting down your total fat intake will reduce your calorie intake and will make it easier for you to get slim — and stay slim. And reducing your intake of saturated fat will dramatically improve your health and reduce your susceptibility to a wide range of disorders (particularly heart disease and high blood pressure).

It is essential to have some fat in your diet in order to stay healthy and fit. There are two obvious reasons why your body needs some fat.

First, essential vitamins such as A and D are soluble in fat. If your diet doesn't include any fat then you may become short in these vitamins.

Second, some polyunsaturated fatty acids are needed for the maintenance of your cell membranes and for the production of vital substances such as prostaglandins.

But it is desperately important that you try to keep your intake of fat to a minimum. If you eat too much fat — and an ordinary, modern, Western diet will almost certainly contain too much fat — then you will run a risk of developing clogged arteries, heart disease and high blood pressure.

Three ways in which a low fat diet will improve your health

1. Fat is rich in calories. If you eat a diet which contains a lot of fat then there is a big chance that you will become obese — and you will subsequently have difficulty in losing that excess weight. Eating a low fat diet will make it easier for you to get slim — and stay slim.

2. If you eat a diet which contains too much saturated fat then you will run a real risk of developing potentially deadly heart disease. A

low fat diet won't make you immune from heart disease — but it will reduce your susceptibility to this type of illness.

3. A high fat diet will increase your risk of developing cancer. Keeping down your intake of fat will cut your risk of developing cancer.

Ten easy ways to reduce the amount of fat you eat

1. Don't fry or roast food. Grill, steam, poach, casserole, bake or boil — but don't fry or roast unless you absolutely must. If you do fry then use a non-stick pan so that you don't have to add lots of extra fat to whatever it is that you are cooking.

2. Drink skimmed or semi-skimmed milk rather than the full fat variety.

3. Avoid butter and margarine (which contain a lot of saturated fat) and use low fat spreads instead. You will find it easier to be more sparing with fatty spreads if you make an effort to buy bread which you really like. Good bread doesn't need a layer of fat to make it palatable.

4. If you must eat meat (which isn't good for your health) then eat only lean meat; avoid red meat whenever you can (because red meat is often rich in hidden or invisible fat); cut off visible fat before cooking or eating, and after grilling or cooking meat on a rack (so that the fat drips out), throw the fat away rather than try to find a use for it in the kitchen.

5. Use oil which is rich in polyunsaturates and which contains few saturates, instead of a hard fat, when you are baking.

6. When making chips out of potatoes cut them thickly (because they will soak up less fat), make sure that the fat or oilyou use is very hot before you add the chips (they will soak up less of the fat if it is very hot) and dry them on kitchen paper after you have cooked them in order to remove any excess oil.

7. If you must buy cream buy single cream rather than double cream. It is often possible to replace cream in recipes with yoghurt.

8. Try to choose low fat cheese, yoghurt, salad dressings and other products when you are shopping.

9. Add herbs rather than butter to vegetables when you have cooked them. Vegetables don't need to have butter added to them if they have been properly cooked.

10. Try to use less fat in cooking. Experiment with low fat recipes.

How much fat is there in the food you eat?

It is often difficult to find out how much fat there is in particular foods. And it is often terribly easy to eat foods which contain a lot of fat without realising it. This specially produced list below is designed to help solve that problem. It may contain a few surprises.

Remember that the figures on this list are only approximate figures intended to be used as a general guide. And remember that if you cook in additional fat the effective fat content of the food you are cooking will rise — often dramatically.

To calculate the percentage of fat in foods which are not on this list look at the calorie list on the package label and divide the number of calories obtained from fat by the total number of calories; then multiply that total by 100 to obtain the percentage.

Almonds 56%

Anchovies 20%

Anchovy, canned, drained 20%

Apple 1%

Apple juice 0%

Apple, baked 0%

Apricot 0%

Artichoke 0%

Asparagus 0%

Aubergine 0%

Avocado pear 22%

Bacon, back fried 44%

Bacon, back grilled 35%

Bacon, streaky 38%

Baked beans 1 %

Banana 0%

Beans, green 0%

Beans, kidney 1%

Beans, lentils 0%

Beans, lima 0%

Beans, pinto 0%

Beef, minced 26%

Beef, roast 34%

Beef suet 95%

Beefburger 27%

Beer 0%

Beetroot 0%

Biscuits, chocolate (digestives) 24%

Biscuits, chocolate chip 20%

Biscuits, cream sandwich 26%

Biscuits, digestive 20%

Biscuits, macaroon 23%

Biscuits, plain 17%

Black pudding 25%

Blackberries 0%

Blackcurrant drink 0%

Blackcurrants 0%

Bran 6%

Bran flakes 2%

Bran wheat 5%

Brazil nuts 61 %

Bread, brown 2%

Bread, Currant 8%

Bread, English muffin 2%

Bread, French stick 3%

Bread, granary 3%

Bread roll (white) 7%

Bread, rye 2%

Bread, soda 3%

Bread, wheatgerm 2%

Bread, white 2%

Bread, white, fried 32%

Bread, white, toasted 1 %

Bread, wholemeal 3%

Broad beans 1 %

Broccoli 0%

Brown sauce 0%

Brussels sprouts 0%

Butter 82%

Cabbage 0%

Carrot 0%

Cashew nuts, roasted, unsalted 46%

Cauliflower 0%

Caviar, black 16%

Celery 0%

Chapatti 1%

Cheese, Austrian smoked 22%

Cheese, Blue Brie 38%

Cheese, Boursin 42%

Cheese, Brie 27%

Cheese, Caerphilly 31%

Cheese, Camembert 23%

Cheese, Cheddar 33%

Cheese, Cheshire 31%

Cheese, Cottage (low fat) 2%

Cheese, Cream 47%

Cheese, Danish Blue 30%

Cheese, Double Gloucester 34%

Cheese, Edam 28%

Cheese, Emmenthal 30%

Cheese, Feta 20%

Cheese, Fromage Frais 7%

Cheese, Gorgonzola 34%

Cheese, Gouda 31%

Cheese, Gruyere 32%

Cheese, Lancashire 31 %

Cheese, Leicester 34%

Cheese, Marscarpone 46%

Cheese, Mozarella 21 %

Cheese, Parmesan 33%

Cheese, Roquefort 31%

Cheese, Stilton, blue 35%

Cheese, Stilton, white 31 %

Cheese, Wensleydale 31%

Cherries 0%

Chestnuts 3%

Chickpeas 2%

Chicken, dark meat, no skin 6%

Chicken, light meat, no skin 5%

Chicken, roast 14%

Chicory 0%

Chillies 1%

Chinese leaves 0%

Chocolate bar, milk 30%

Chocolate bar, plain 30%

Chocolate bar with nuts 26%

Chocolate drink 6%

Chutney 0%

Cider 0%

Cockles, shelled 1%

Cocoa 20%

Coconut, shredded 35%

Cod, steamed 1%

Cod, grilled 1%

Cod fillet in batter 10%

Cod's roe 4%

Coffee 0%

Cola drink 0%

Coleslaw 5%

Coley, raw 1%

Corn, canned, cream style 1 %

Corn, canned 1%

Corn on the cob, fresh 0%

Cornflakes 1%

Corned beef 33%

Courgettes 0%

Crabmeat 5%

Cranberry sauce 0%

Cream, aerosol spray 32%

Cream, clotted 64%

Cream, double 48%

Cream, Fraiche, Half fat 10%

Cream, Fraiche 27%

Cream, half cream 14%

Cream, single 20%

Cream, sour 20%

Cream, whipping 39%

Cream crackers 16%

Crispbread 2%

Crumpet 1%

Cucumber 0%

Custard 4%

Danish pastry 26%

Dates, dried 1%

Duck, roasted without skin 10%

Duck's egg 14%

Egg, boiled 11%

Egg, fried 19%

Egg, omelette 16%

Figs, dried 0%

Figs, fresh 0%

Fish cakes (fried) 11%

Fish fingers (fried) 13%

Fish paste 10%

Flour, white 1%

Flour, wholemeal 2%

Gammon rasher 12%

Garlic 0%

Gin, whisky, vodka, brandy 0%

Ginger ale 0%

Goat's milk 5%

Golden syrup 0%

Goose 22%

Gooseberries 0%

Grapefruit 0%

Grapefruit juice, unsweetened 0%

Grapes, black 0%

Grapes, white 0%

Gravy (meat juices, fat, flour and stock) 9%

Haddock fillet, smoked 1%

Halibut, steamed 16%

Ham 26%

Hazel nuts 36%

Herring, grilled 13%

Herring, pickled 18%

Herring, raw 18%

Herring, rollmop 10%

Honey 0%

Horseradish sauce 8%

Hot dog sausages 25%

Ice cream 16%

Jam 0%

Jelly 0%

Kidney, fried 6%

Kipper, baked 45%

Kipper grilled 11%

Kiwi fruit 1%

Lager 0%

Lamb chop, grilled 22%

Lamb leg, roasted 24%

Lamb shoulder, roasted 29%

Lard 99%

Leeks 0%

Lemon 0%

Lemon curd 5%

Lemonade 0%

Lentils 1%

Lettuce 1%

Liver, lamb's, fried 14%

Liver, pig's, braised 8%

Lobster 3%

Low fat spread 40%

Luncheon meat 27%

Lychees 0%

Macadamia nuts 73%

Mackerel 11 %

Mackerel flesh, raw 16%

Mackerel, fillet, smoked 13%

Malt loaf 3%

Malted milk drink 7%

Mandarin oranges 0%

Mango 0%

Margarine, low fat 40%

Margarine, very low fat 25%

Margarine, full fat, 81 %

Marmalade 0%

Marrow 0%

Marzipan 25%

Mayonnaise 79%

Meat pie 24%

Melon, cantaloupe 0%

Melon, honey dew 0%

Milk, condensed 9%

Milk, evaporated 9%

Milk, fresh semi-skimmed 2%

Milk, fresh skimmed 1 %

Milk, fresh whole 4%

Milk, skimmed, powder 1%

Mince pie 21 %

Mincemeat 4%

Mints 1%

Mixed vegetables (frozen) 0%

Molasses 0%

Mousse (fruit) 7%

Muesli 8%

Mushrooms, fried 22%

Mushrooms, raw 1%

Mussels 2%

Mustard and cress 0%

Mustard 8%

Nectarine 0%

Noodles, egg 2%

Oil, coconut 97%

Oil, corn 97%

Oil, olive 96%

Oil, peanut 96%

Oil, soybean 97%

Oil, sunflower 97%

Okra 0%

Olives (in brine) 11 %

Onion, fried 33%

Onion, raw 0%

Orange 0%

Orange juice, unsweetened 0%

Orange squash 0%

Oysters 1%

Pancake 7%

Parsley 0%

Parsnips 0%

Passion fruit 0%

Pasta, boiled 1 %

Peach, fresh 0%

Peaches, tinned 0%

Peanut butter 51%

Peanuts, salted 49%

Pear 0%

Peas, frozen 0%

Peas, tinned 0%

Pecans 74%

Pepper, green 0%

Pepper, red 0%

Pickle 0%

Pilchards 5%

Pineapple juice 0%

Pineapple, fresh 0%

Pineapple, tinned 0%

Pitta bread 1%

Plaice, steamed 2%

Plum 0%

Popcorn (no salt or fat) 5%

Pork chop 18%

Pork leg, roasted 32%

Pork pie 29%

Pork, spareribs 39%

Porridge with water 1%

Port 0%

Potatoes, boiled 0%

Potatoes, deep fried chips 40%

Potato, jacket 0%

Potatoes, oven chips 8%

Potatoes, roasted 5%

Potatoes, sweet, baked 0%

Prawns 2%

Prunes 1%

Quiche 28%

Rabbit 5%

Radishes 0%

Raisins 0%

Raspberries 0%

Ratatouille 6%

Red wine 0%

Rhubarb (stewed) 0%

Rice, brown, boiled 1%

Rice, white, boiled 0%

Runner beans 0%

Salad dressing: French 39%

Salad dressing: French, low cal 4%

Salad dressing: Italian 60%

Salad dressing: Italian, low cal 5%

Salad dressing: mayonnaise, low calorie 12%

Salad dressing: mayonnaise: 75%

Salami 47%

Salmon, fresh 13%

Salmon, tinned 8%

Sardines 14%

Sausages, beef, grilled 21%

Sausages, pork, grilled 30%

Scampi 21%

Scotch egg 21%

Sesame seeds, dry, hulled 55%

Sherry 0%

Shortbread 26%

Smoked haddock 1%

Smoked salmon 4%

Soy sauce 1%

Soybean curd (tofu) 6%

Spinach 1%

Sponge pudding 16%

Spring greens 0%

Squid 1%

Steak, grilled 6%

Steak and kidney pie 21 %

Steak pudding 12%

Stock cube 3%

Strawberries 0%

Stuffing, sage and onion 0%

Sugar, demerara 0%

Sugar, muscavado 0%

Sugar, white 0%

Sultanas 0%

Sunflower seeds 48%

Swede 0%

Sweet potato 1 %

Sweetcorn 1%

Sweets, boiled 0%

Swiss roll 5%

Syrup, cane and maple 0%

Taco shell, fried tortilla 19%

Tangerine 0%

Taramasalata 46%

Tartar sauce 59%

Tea 0%

Tinned fruit salad 0%

Toffee apple 0%

Toffees 17%

Tomato, fried 6%

Tomato juice 0%

Tomato paste 0%

Tomato puree 0%

Tomato, raw 0%

Tomato soup 3%

Tomatoes, tinned 0%

Tonic water 0%

Treacle 0%

Tripe, stewed 4%

Trout 5%

Tuna fish tinned in oil 22%

Turkey, roast 10%

Turnip 0%

Veal 28%

Vegetable soup 1 %

Venison 6%

Vinegar 0%

Walnuts 52%

Water biscuits 13%

Water chestnuts 1 %

Watercress 0%

Watermelon 0%

White wine 0%

Whitebait 48%

Wine, dessert (port, madeira, sweet sherry) 0%

Wine, table (burgundy, rose, white, dry sherry) 0%

Yam 0%

Yeast extract (Marmite) 0%

Yoghurt, fruit (low fat) 1 %

Yoghurt, plain (low fat) 1 %

Yoghurt, soya 2%

CHAPTER EIGHTEEN

101 SUPERFOODS

Finding out exactly what you should eat isn't quite so easy. The truth is shrouded in mystery and confusion – much of created, quite deliberately, on behalf of vested interests, by lobbyists, advertising agencies and public relations groups.

The far reaching tentacles of the big food companies are as powerful as those of the big drug companies. Finding the truth is made particularly difficult by the fact that many newspapers, magazines and journals readily publish material they are given by companies with products to sell. Television and radio are, of course, just as likely to publicise these commercial messages disguised as independent news items.

Frequently, undue emphasis is placed on small — often almost irrelevant bits and pieces of scientific information — which are fed to the media because they help to build up and strengthen some hidden agenda. Too many observers (by which I mean editors, journalists and commentators) fail to analyse the information which appears; seemingly ignorant of the fact that an overview is necessary if any information is going to be put into perspective and used effectively.

Hyperbole and exaggeration used to be the preserve of the tabloid newspapers. These days they are everyday tools for broadsheet journalists and for just about everyone working in television and radio.

Sponsorship is widespread and often subtle, and this can make it difficult to decide exactly what is true and what isn't. Hidden agendas are sometimes well hidden, sometimes hidden only a little and sometimes not hidden at all.

I have prepared a list of the 101 healthiest, tastiest and very best foods in the world. These are foods that don't just taste good and look good - they will provide you with a massive amount of protection against cancer and heart disease, they will boost your immune system and they help reduce your susceptibility to infection.

And whether they agree or disagree with the contents of this list you can be confident that no one has sponsored this list.

Naturally, you don't have to limit yourself to the foods on this list which I have compiled as a starting point: a healthy basis for any good, well-balanced, diet.

The list will, I hope, also help the many readers who have written to me explaining that they plan to become vegetarian (or vegan) but confessing that they really don't know what to eat.

I've arranged this list in alphabetical order — partly because I think it will make it easier to use, and partly because I didn't want to print a list that suggested that any one particular food was 'number one'.

To make the list more accessible I haven't listed all the specific nutrients and health giving ingredients these foods contain but have simply given a very brief summary of the main qualities of individual foods.

Foods which contain anti-oxidants (such as vitamins C and E, the mineral selenium and beta-carotene, which are converted in the human body to vitamin A) help prevent cancer and heart disease and reduce susceptibility to infection.

My recommended healthy diet would contain a good and varied selection of foods from this list.

1. Alfalfa sprouts

Low in protein and don't contain much in the way of minerals or vitamins but they are also low in fat, calories and sodium. They are a tasty filler for salads and sandwiches.

2. Almonds

Rich in vitamin E (an anti-oxidant), plus calcium and protein. (But watch out: they also contain a high proportion of fat.)

3. Apples

Will help strengthen your immune system. Apples contain lots of fibre and plenty of vitamins. Easily obtainable and relatively inexpensive apples make a great snack and an excellent ingredient for pies and crumbles. But try to buy apples which are not covered with a wax coating to preserve them. More natural apples may not have the 'sheen' of a waxed apple but they will be better for you.

4. Apricots

Like all orange-coloured fruits and vegetables apricots are packed with the anti-oxidant beta-carotene which helps protect against cancer. Apricots are also full of fibre. Dried apricots make an excellent snack food. (Buy organic dried apricots not the bright orange ones.)

5. Artichoke

May help reduce blood fat and cholesterol levels and may help with liver, gall bladder and digestive problems.

6. Asparagus

Has a diuretic effect and is also believed to be useful in the treatment of nausea, heartburn and hiatus hernia.

7. Aubergine (eggplant)

In South East Asia some people use it to treat stomach cancer. Not a food to fry because it absorbs huge amounts of fat.

8. Avocado Pear

Because it grows in clusters rather than singly the avocado should officially be classed as a berry rather than a pear. Theavocado tree yields more food per acre than any other tree crop and before humans started eating them they were popular with animals as varied as dinosaurs, giant sloths and jaguars.

The avocado contains a rich mixture of nutrients — 14 minerals (including copper, iron, calcium, potassium and magnesium), 11 vitamins and a lot of protein. An additional point in their favour is that the avocado is low in sodium. This makes them good for individuals who are on a low salt diet.

The oil content of the avocado can be quite high. It is believed that the avocado also contains special anti-bacterial and anti-fungal ingredients. Some say the avocado has anticancer properties.

9. Baked beans

Excellent source of fibre.

10. Bananas

Prepacked in a moisture and bug proof wrapping (so environmentally friendly and so biodegradable that you can quickly turn it into compost) that ensures the fruit inside arrives with you clean, fresh and uncontaminated, bananas are packed with vitamins and minerals and fibre and carbohydrate and very low in fat. Bananas, which are rich in potas-sium and contain a useful quantity of vitamin C, make an excellent snacking food for picnics or people who are travelling.

11. Bean sprouts

A good source of vitamins B and C. Also contain protein.

12. Beans

A good source of potassium and folate. May help prevent or treat anaemia. May help reduce the risk of heart disease. High in fibre and protein. Pulses are usually low in fat.

13. Beetroot

Good source of folate and iron.

14. Bilberry (aka blueberry)

Believed to help improve the circulation and to counteracturinary tract infections. Bilberries have anti-oxidant, anti-inflammatory and anti-infective effects.

15. Blackberries

Excellent low fat source of vitamin E.

16. Blackcurrant

An excellent source of vitamin C. (Weight for weight blackcurrants contain four times as much vitamin C as oranges.) Moreover the blackcurrant retains its vitamin C content well. Blackcurrants contain anthocyanins which are anti-inflammatory and which inhibit bacteria such as E.coli, holidaying merrily among the villae of the intestinal riviera.

17. Bread

Not for nothing is bread traditionally known as the 'staff of life'. Wholemeal bread is particularly good for you. Rich in fibre and vitamins and minerals wholemeal bread should play a large part in any healthy diet. A 'honey on wholemeal bread' sandwich makes an excellent quick snack.

18. Broad beans

A good source of protein and soluble fibre.

19. Broccoli

Several studies have shown that vegetables such as broccoli can help to stop you getting cancer. Other vegetables which have the same apparently magical 'superfood' effect include cauliflower, cabbage and Brussels sprouts. These vegetables are believed to help prevent cancer because they contain compounds called indole glycosinolates (known for short as IGs). Cancers which may be prevented — or slowed — by these vegetables include cancers of the breast, colon and stomach.

However, cooking or even slight steaming seems to reduce the anti-cancer quality of these vegetables which seem to be most powerful when eaten raw. Cutting the vegetables into fairly small pieces seems to increase their anti-cancer power.

20. Brussels sprouts

Contain anti-oxidants and other substances which provide protection against cancer.

21. Cabbage

Contains substances which provide protection against cancer.

22. Carrots

Contain anti-oxidants. A great, healthy snack food. I often stuff a carrot and an apple in my bag when travelling. Full of fibre, vitamins and minerals, carrots are excellent cooked or eaten raw. Most children enjoy chewing on a raw carrot — it is an excellent and healthy alternative to a biscuit or bar of chocolate.

23. Cauliflower

Contains anti-oxidants and other substances which provide protection against cancer.

24. Celeriac

A good source of potassium. When eaten raw (e.g. in salads) it is also a good source of vitamin C.

25. Cherries

Contain potassium and vitamin C.

26. Chestnuts

High in carbohydrates and fibre but, unusually for nuts, low in fat. Brazil nuts, walnuts and hazelnuts have more than twenty times as much fat as chestnuts. Contain vitamin E and vitamin B6.

27. Chickpeas

Will help reduce cholesterol levels. Impecunious Indians who live on a chickpea diet have low blood cholesterol. Contain anti-oxidants.

28. Chillies

Chilli pepper may help desensitise the airways and may help stop an asthma attack. By having a mildly irritant effect onthe stomach chillies may also stimulate the stomach to defend itself against more serious threats — and may help to protect against damage and the development of ulcers. The substance which gives chillies their fierce flavour is capsaicin which is an anti-oxidant which helps provide protection against cancer.

29. Corn

Contains protein, iron, zinc and potassium. Low in sodium. The Tarahumara Indians of Mexico live on a diet of corn and beans. High blood cholesterol and artery clogging and their fateful consequences are virtually unknown among these people. Contain anti-oxidants.

30. Courgettes (Zucchini)

A type of small marrow and a useful source of vitamin C and folate. Also a good source of beta-carotene. Most of the nutrients are stored in the skins, which are edible.

31. Cranberry

Widely used as a home remedy in the treatment of bladder, kidney and urinary tract infection. Recent research has shown that cranberries contain something which prevents bacteria from multiplying in the urinary tract. The only other fruit to have a similar effect is the bilberry (aka blueberry).

32. Cress

A cruciferous vegetable which can help prevent the development of cancer. Rich in vitamins and minerals. May help prevent anaemia and heart disease.

33. Dates

Dried dates are rich in potassium and a good source of many other nutrients too (including iron).

34. Fennel

Toasted fennel seeds are chewed in India to prevent indigestion and bad breath. Alternatively the seeds can be used to make a tea which helps digestive problems including flatulenceand colic. Fennel seeds should be avoided during pregnancy.

35. Figs

Rich in potassium and fibre. Also contain pectin which can help lower blood cholesterol levels.

36. Garlic

There is a growing amount of evidence available now to show that if it is eaten regularly garlic will help to reduce your chances of having a heart attack. Garlic has been used for thousands of years as a flavouring and as a preventive medicine. It seems that it can reduce the level of fat and cholesterol in the blood and also help prevent blood clotting. These factors mean that garlic may well help to prevent heart disease. Certainly, the evidence is powerful enough not to be ignored. The value of garlic is enhanced by the fact that unlike many modern drugs is contains no significant side effects (unless you count the antisocial effect of the smell on your breath as a significant side effect). I believe that garlic, onions, chives, leeks and shallots will all provide protection against cancer and infection as well as against heart disease.

37. Ginger

Helps relieve nausea, flatulence and indigestion. May stimulate the circulation and prevent blood clots. May also relieve rheumatism. Ginger keeps many of its properties when dried.

38. Grapefruit

Packed with vitamins (especially vitamin C) and rich in fibre. Will help strengthen the immune system. Contains anti-oxidants. Pink grapefruit contains lycopene which helps provide protection against cancer (particularly prostate cancer) and heart disease.

39. Grapes

Grapes contain ellagic acid which may help prevent cancer developing. (Cherries and strawberries contain the same substance).

40. Hazelnuts

Contain vitamin E (an anti-oxidant) plus vitamins B1 and B6. Also contain protein. The downside is a high fat content.

41. Honey

Although it is sugar with one or two added vitamins and minerals honey does seem to have some mysterious and almost 'magical' qualities. Honey is being prescribed more and more often by doctors.

Theoretically, honey shouldn't be of any special value. But surgeons have found that if they spread honey onto infected wounds and burns then healing takes place much faster. It seems that honey helps to clean the tissues and conquer the infection.

Second, doctors have found that honey kills dangerous bugs like salmonella, cholera and escherichia coli quickly and efficiently.

Third, it has been shown that honey is better at killing many of the bugs that cause urinary infection than some powerful, modern drugs such as penicillin.

Fourth, research has shown that children suffering from gastro-enteritis seem to get better quicker if given honey to eat.

No one seems to know just why honey works so well. But there seems little doubt that honey is one of the great 'magical mystery' foods.

42. Hummus

Contains chickpeas, sesame seeds, garlic, coriander seeds, lemon juice and olive oil. It is, consequently, packed with goodness (but buy a low fat version).

43. Kale

A very good source of vitamin C and beta-carotene. Also, like other deep green vegetables, kale is a good source of calcium and iron. It also contains compounds which may provide protection against cancer.

44. Kidney beans

A good source of protein. Contains potassium, zinc and iron. But be careful: raw or undercooked kidney beans can cause serious food poisoning.

45. Lentils

A good source of protein, fibre, minerals and vitamins.

46. Lettuce

Lettuce (and other salad greens) provides protection against cancer (particularly cancer of the stomach). Also contains the anti-oxidant vitamins C and E. A good source of iron. May also aid digestion.

47. Lime

May help to reduce cancer risk. May also help to prevent infection. A good source of potassium.

48. Linseed

A good source of omega 3 fatty acids which lower the risk of colorectal cancer by reducing the amount of prostaglandin in the bowel. May aid digestion and prevent constipation. May also help prevent breast cancer and may help ease menopausal symptoms.

49. Lychees

An excellent source of vitamin C.

50. Mango

A useful source of vitamins C and E when raw. Also contain iron. A good source of carotene — particularly when ripe.

51. Melon

Watermelon contains lycopene which helps provide protection against cancer (particularly prostate cancer) and heart disease. Melon with orange flesh (such as cantaloupe) is rich in carotene.

52. Mushrooms

Contain protein, vitamins and minerals but are low in fat and calories. Rich in potassium, iron and niacin. Some varieties may discourage the development of cancer. Try to buy field picked mushrooms rather than specially grown mushrooms if you can — they taste better.

53. Mustard

Mustard (commonly grown with cress) may help prevent cancer and heart disease.

54. Oats

Whether you eat them in porridge or in specially made bread, buns or biscuits you'll benefit enormously by increasing your consumption of oats. Oat bran contains protein, carbohydrate and vitamin B — and more useful fibre than any other food. A regular addition of oat bran to your diet will help you lose weight and stay slim. Plus, oat bran will also help to reduce your blood cholesterol level and, therefore, reduce your chances of having a heart attack or a stroke.

55. Olive oil

Cold pressed extra virgin olive oil is a good source of vitamin E.

56. Olives

A good source of vitamin E.

57. Onions

Onions, chives, leeks and shallots may all provide protection against cancer, infection and heart disease.

58. Orange

Oranges, like bananas, come in their own environmentally-friendly wrapper (even if you throw it down it soon rots). Oranges contain slightly less fibre than bananas but they are packed with vitamins (especially vitamin C) and minerals. A genuine, fresh fruit salad which consists of orange, banana and apple will make a cheap, tasty and healthy pudding.

59. Papaya (pawpaw)

Contains carotene and vitamin C and, when raw, an enzyme which digests protein.

60. Parsley

An enormously underestimated food which often ends up being used as a sprig of decoration on the side of the plate — and then not even eaten! Parsley contains essential protein and useful vitamins and minerals,

61. Parsnip

A useful source of starch and fibre and of vitamins C and E.

62. Passion fruit

Contain vitamin C.

63. Pasta

Available in many different forms — as spaghetti, lasagna, tagliatelle, macaroni etc. — pasta is the athlete's favourite food. Professional cyclists, athletes and other sportsmen and women eat pasta at most of their main meals — particularly on the night before a big event. Pasta contains a good quantity of complex carbohydrate and a lot of fibre but is low in fat. It is cheap, easy and quick to cook and very filling.

64. Peaches

Rich in vitamin C. Dried peaches contain a good deal of potassium.

65. Pears

A good source of natural sugar. Contain some vitamins.

66. Peas

Rich in vitamin B1 and a good source of vitamin C. Contain fibre, protein, phosphorus and folate.

67. Peppers

An excellent source of vitamin C. Red peppers contain more vitamin C than green peppers and are also an excellent source of beta-carotene. Although they are extremely low in calories peppers are among the most nutritious foods you can buy.

68. Pine nuts

Contain iron, manganese, magnesium and zinc — as well as vitamin B1 and vitamin E (an anti-oxidant). Also contain protein. Downside is a high fat content.

69. Pineapple

Contain anti-oxidants.

70. Pinto beans

High in protein and fibre and low in fat.

71. Plums

Contain vitamin E and potassium.

72. Pomegranate

A good source of vitamin C.

73. Potato

Potatoes are almost certainly the most under-valued food in the world and the most mistreated. Potatoes are rich in vitamins (particularly vitamin C) and are an excellent foodstuff. To get the most out of them you should try to eat your potatoes in their jackets.

If you eat potatoes as chips keep the fat down by cutting them thickly, making sure that the oil you use (preferably vegetable oil high in polyunsaturates and low in saturates) is sizzling hot before you add the chips and drying the chips on a piece of kitchen towel before you serve them.

When cooked properly and wisely potatoes make an excellent food. When cooked unwisely the goodness in potatoes can be destroyed and the amount of fat they contain can be dramatically increased,

74. Prunes

Contain vitamins and minerals as well as heaps of fibre. Good to add to breakfast cereals or salads. Gentle laxative effect.

75. Pumpkin

Packed with cancer preventing beta-carotene plus plenty of other vitamins and minerals — and fibre too. Pumpkin seeds, which contain zinc, are widely used to help prevent (and treat) prostate enlargement.

76. Radishes

Useful source of vitamin C.

77. Raspberries

Rich in vitamin C.

78. Redcurrant

Rich in vitamin G and potassium.

79. Rhubarb

A good source of potassium.

80. Rice

Brown rice contains anti-oxidants. Rice bran may help reduce the risk of bowel cancer. A good source of starch.

81. Runner beans

Contain iron, folate and vitamin C.

82. Seaweed

Contains beta-carotene and B vitamins as well as many minerals. Most types of seaweed are a good source of iodine.

83. Sesame seeds

Contain vitamin E and calcium.

84. Soya beans

Soya beans are almost certainly one of the world's most valuable crops. They are packed with protein and contain anti-oxidants. If farmers around the world grew soya beans instead of breeding animals there would be no need for anyone anywhere to be hungry. Soya is used in the preparation of a vast array of different products which include milk and yoghurt substitutes as well as textured vegetable protein — also known as TVP Soya is an enormously flexible foodstuff but it is important to remember that the basic ingredients for a healthy diet are vegetables, fruit and whole grains.

85. Spinach

Popeye was right! Spinach is rich in vitamins, minerals, fibre and protein — and low in calories and fat. The usual mistake is to overcook spinach so that it becomes soggy and tasteless (as well as less valuable nutritionally). If spinach is bought fresh and properly cooked it will be both tastier and better for you. Can be used raw in salads.

86. Squash (Winter)

Pumpkins and other winter squash are a good source of beta-carotene.

87. Strawberries

Contains anti-oxidants. One of the richest sources of vitamin C.

88. Sunflower oil

Rich in vitamin E.

89. Sunflower seeds

Rich in zinc.

90. Swedes

May help to prevent cancer. A good source of vitamin C.

91. Sweet potato (yam)

Contains anti-oxidants.

92. Tea

A gentle stimulant which also supplies an anti-oxidant which may lower the risk of cancer and heart disease. But drink in moderation. (No more than two or three cups a day.)

93. Tomatoes

Contain lycopene which helps provide protection against cancer — particularly prostate cancer. Men who eat tomato-basedfoods (particularly tomato ketchup, canned tomatoes, tomato soup, tomato-based spaghetti sauce and the tomato sauce used in preparing pizza) are less likely to develop prostate cancer. Lycopene may also protect against heart disease and other cancers. It is the heat processing which seems to increase the availability of lycopene in tomatoes. So frying tomatoes should also increase their lycopene availability.

94. Turnip

A good source of fibre and vitamin C.

95. Walnut

Help lower blood cholesterol and may help prevent heart disease. Rich in essential fatty acids which are vital for tissue growth and development.

96. Watercress

Although it is rich in vitamins and minerals watercress is virtually calorie free. It makes an excellent addition to any salad and is much under-utilised by chefs and sandwich makers.

97. Wheat

The consumption of wheat fibre is linked to a lower cancer risk (particularly breast cancer). May help relieve menopausal symptoms and prevent heart disease.

98. Wheatgerm

The most nutrient rich part of wheat. Provides vitamins B and E.

99. Wine

Red wine drinkers seem to have a reduced incidence of heart disease. Moderation is the key. One or two glasses a day seem ideal. Red wine is also believed to have an anti-oxidant effect (and may provide some protection against viruses too).

100. Wholegrains

Wholegrain barley, buckwheat, maize and rye may help prevent heart disease, high blood pressure, diabetes and some cancers.

101 Yoghurt

Natural yoghurt (not the sweetened, fruit and calorie filled variety) is really good for you. It is high in protein and calcium and a good source of iron and some of the vitamins in the B group. Yoghurt contains lactobacilli which compete with and oust numerous infections — including thrush.

Everyone should try to eat natural yoghurt regularly. Women who are suffering from thrush can often ease their symptoms by dipping a tampon in natural yoghurt before inserting it. Sufferers from irritable bowel syndrome sometimes find that they benefit after eating yoghurt (soya yoghurt is now increasingly available for those who wish or need to avoid dairy produce). Watch out because some yoghurts contain many additives which you might not want to eat.

CHAPTER NINETEEN

OVERWEIGHT

Overweight caused by overeating is the biggest cause of death in the Western world. At least one in three of us needs to lose weight. Being fat doesn't just make people miserable — and make it difficult for them to wear the clothes they'd like to wear — it makes diseases as varied as asthma, gout, diabetes, high blood pressure and arthritis worse, and it *kills* people.

If you weigh too much you are more likely to have a stroke or suffer from diabetes. Eczema, varicose veins, piles, gall stones and hernias are all associated with obesity. People who are overweight are more likely to face extra risks if they need to have surgery (because having an anaesthetic is more dangerous if you are overweight) and women who are fat face extra difficulties if they get pregnant.

In addition excess fat makes many lives miserable, causes depression and makes crippling diseases such as asthma and arthritis considerably worse.

Heart disease of all kinds is made much worse when patients weigh too much. In many cases heart disease is brought on because of obesity. The fatter you are the greater the burden will be on your heart.

Diabetes mellitus is now so common that 2% of the population have it. And the number of diabetics is doubling every ten years. Many patients become diabetic because they eat too much. Thousands of cases of diabetes could be prevented if people ate less fattening food. Overweight people are far more likely to get diabetes than people of average or below average weight. Diabetes is caused by a malfunction in the pancreatic gland — the gland that produces the hormone insulin. Insulin helps the body make proper use of carbohydrates in your food.

Many of those who develop diabetes — and this is particularly true of those who develop the disease in late adulthood — can get rid of the signs and symptoms of the disease by dieting, losing weight and carefully controlling their food intake. (All this should, of course, be done under medical supervision.)

Losing excess weight will help your body in hundreds of different ways. Even your feet will benefit. An average sized pair of feet provide their owner with less than 50 square inches of support. You can get some idea of the sort of strain there is on your feet by trying to hold a bag of flour on the tip of one finger. Losing weight dramatically reduces the pressure on your feet and makes bunions, corns and similar problems far less likely.

Here are some of the specific ways in which being overweight can affect your health:

YOUR JOINTS

Fat people are far more likely to suffer from arthritis and rheumatism. Because they have more weight to carry around, their joints and ligaments creak under the strain. The knees are often the first to give way. Losing excess weight won't repair the damage that has already been done to your joints; but it will dramatically reduce the incidence of future problems. Arthritis and backache sufferers who are overweight will usually suffer from less pain — and become more mobile — if they lose weight.

YOUR HEART

Your heart has to supply the rest of your body with fresh blood — delivering oxygen and then taking away the waste products. The bigger your body is the harder your heart has to work. An average heart beats seventy times a minute and if your heart has to work 20% harder (because you are 20% overweight) the strain will tell. If your heart beats 70 times a minute then it will beat 4,200 times an hour; 100,800 times a day; 705,600 times a week; 36,691,200 times a year and an astonishing 2,568,384,000 times in an average lifetime. Add another 20% to that total and you can see the difference it makes. A small 1500 cc motor car engine may work very well when put in a small car body but if the same engine is put into a bus it will soon show real signs of overstrain. Getting rid of your excess weight will ensure that the strain on your heart is reduced — and in the long run that means that your chances of suffering from heart trouble will fall significantly.

YOUR SKIN

Because fat acts as a sort of insulation — keeping the body warm — overweight people sweat a great deal more than thin people when the weather is hot. To this must be added the fact that fat people tend to have deep skin creases in which the sweat can accumulate. These skin creases are difficult to keep clean and dry — so fungal infections are commonplace. Women who are overweight often find that their abdominal skin creases and the areas around their groins and under their breasts are particularly likely to cause problems and eczema or dermatitis often develop.

Losing weight means that fat disappears but if the skin has been stretched for a long period of time the skin folds may not disappear and when this happens surgery may be needed to remove the excess skin.

YOUR BLOOD PRESSURE

Blood normally travels around your body under pressure — much in the same way that water travels through a hose-pipe under pressure. If you use a longer hose then you'll need more pressure to push the water through as quickly. And if your body gets bigger then your blood pressure will need to increase to make sure that all parts of your body continue to receive a good blood supply. When blood pressure rises there is a danger that a blood vessel will be unable to take the strain and may burst. If you lose your excess weight then your blood pressure should fall — and you will be less likely to have a stroke.

YOUR LUNGS

Your chest is permanently expanding and contracting as air is sucked into and forced out of your lungs. If your chest wall is thick with fat breathing becomes more difficult. This will become particularly noticeable on slight exertion and explains why overweight people often appear to be short of breath. The shortage of fresh air getting into the lungs means that the blood is short of oxygen — and that means that the heart has to work even harder to keep the tissues supplied. People who are overweight are more likely to suffer from heart disease and from lung disorders such as asthma and bronchitis. Losing excess weight often means that some of the fatty tissue around the lungs disappears — freeing the lungs.

YOUR VEINS

Blood in your legs gets up to your heart through your veins. It is the muscles in your legs which help to squeeze the blood upwards. If you are overweight your muscles will have difficulty in squeezing your veins so your blood will tend to stay where it is — producing swollen or varicose veins. Losing excess weight helps to make sure that this problem doesn't get any worse.

CHAPTER TWENTY

HOW MUCH SHOULD YOU WEIGH?

There is no doubt that the simplest and most reliable way to find out whether or not you are overweight is to weigh yourself.

Unfortunately, it isn't always as easy as it should be to decide from this just how much weight you need to lose. Many of the height weight charts which are in existence are pretty useless. Some of them were devised many years ago when people were much skinnier (and less muscular) than they are today. As a result, the charts seem to suggest that virtually everyone who isn't skeletal needs to lose weight.

I also have grave misgivings about height weight charts which require you to decide whether you are small, medium or large boned before you can use them. It's nigh on impossible to decide this without first stripping off all your flesh but even if it was a practical question it is of relatively little significance because bones don't usually weigh all that much and the difference between large and small bones is a fairly small one.

I have compiled special height weight tables which enable you to compare your weight with the ideal weight for your height. I've given you an ideal weight band — you should try to make sure that your weight falls into this band.

Height/weight chart for women

Instructions

1. Weigh yourself with as few clothes as possible — and no shoes.
2. Measure your height in bare or stockinged feet.
3. You are overweight if your weight falls above your ideal weight band.

Height Weight Band

(ft/in) (st/lb)

4.10 — 7.5-8.5

4.11 — 7.7-8.7

5.0 — 7.9-8.9

5.1 — 7.11-8.11

5.2 — 8.1-9.1

5.3 — 8.4-9.4

5.4 — 8.6-9.6

5.5 — 8.10-9.10

5.6 — 9.0-10.0

5.7 — 9.3-10.3

5.8 — 9.7-10.7

5.9 — 9.10-10.10

5.10 — 10.0-11.0

5.11 — 10.3-11.3

6. 0 — 10.7-11.7

6.1 — 10.9-11.9

6.2 — 10.12-11.12

6.3 — 11.2-12.2

6.4 — 11.5-12.5

NOTE

Ideal weights vary with age and various other factors. But if you weigh more than 14 pounds above the maximum in your Ideal Weight Band then your weight will almost certainly be having an adverse effect on your health.

Height/weight chart for men

Instructions

1. Weigh yourself with as few clothes as possible — and no shoes.

2. Measure your height in bare feet or socks.

3. You are overweight if your weight falls above your ideal weight band.

Height Weight Band
(ft/in) (st/lb)
5.0 — 8.5-9.5
5.1 — 8.6-9.6
5.2 — 8.7-9.7
5.3 — 8.8-9.8
5.4 — 8.11-9.11
5.5 — 9.2-10.2
5.6 — 9.6-10.6
5.7 — 9.10-10.10
5.8 — 10.0-11.0
5.9 — 10.4-11.4
5.10 — 10.8-11.8
5.11 — 10.12-11.12
6. 0 — 11.2-12.2
6.1 — 11.6-12.6
6.2 — 11.10-12.10
6.3 — 12.0-13.0
6.4 — 12.4-13.4
6.5 — 12.8-13.8
6.6 — 13.0-14.0

NOTE

Ideal weights vary with age and various other factors. But if you weigh more than 14 pounds above the maximum in your Ideal

Weight Band then your weight will almost certainly be having an adverse effect on your health.

TRY THE PINCH TEST

When doctors want to find out how much fat there is in someone's body they sometimes use specially designed calipers to do the measuring.

You can use a simple version of this technique yourself. The big advantage of it is that it will enable you to find out which parts of your body contain most fat. (Though you probably already have a pretty good idea of the answer to this question.)

Just pick up a lump of flesh between your thumb and forefinger and see how much space it takes up. If you try this test with the flesh on the back of your hand you will see that there isn't much fat stored there. But if you try the same test around your waist you will find that it is a very different story. Fat deposits vary from site to site around your body.

When you use your thumb and forefinger for this test you are, of course, picking up two layers of skin and two layers of fat. (Since human skin is fairly thin you are effectively holding two thicknesses of body fat.) So, in order to get an idea of the thickness of your body fat at that particular point on your body you have only to halve the distance between your thumb and your forefinger.

You can probably do this measuring yourself. Don't squeeze until it hurts. Just make sure that you have a firm hold on the flesh you want to measure. Then, using a ruler, measure the distance between the skin of your thumb and the skin of your forefinger.

You can do this test all over your body.

If you want to do this test to get an idea of whether or not you are generally fat then the best place for the test is probably the triceps muscle at the back of your upper arm. You can also try measuring the amount of body fat at your waist, on the back of your legs, on your thighs, hips and buttocks.

If the thickness of your skin and under-skin fat exceeds half an inch then there is probably too much fat there. Since the 'pinch test' measures a double thickness of skin and fat this means that anything more than one inch thick means that you have too much fat.

If you can pinch more than an inch then you need to diet.

OR TRY THE MIRROR TEST

Take off all your clothes and stand naked in front of a full length mirror. You should be able to tell whether or not you are overweight — and where the excess weight is — simply by looking at your reflection and being honest with yourself.

OR TRY THE TAPE MEASURE TEST

1. Measure your chest with a tape measure.

2. Measure your waist with a tape measure.

3. If your waist measurement exceeds your chest measurement then you are almost certainly carrying far too much fat around your waist.

OR TRY THE RULER TEST

1. Take off all your clothes.

2. Lie flat on your back.

3. Rest one end of a twelve inch ruler on the bottom edge of your rib cage and the other end on the top end of your pelvis. If the ruler lies firmly on bone (with no flesh touching it in the middle) then you don't have a fat tummy. If, however, the ruler bobs about (particularly if you breathe or laugh) then you probably need to lose weight — and your waist is probably one of the places where you have got most fat stored.

OR TRY THE WAIST AND HIP TEST

Divide your waist measurement by your hip measurement.

If you are a woman and the answer is 0.85 or more then you need to lose weight.

If you are a man and the answer is 1.00 or more then you need to lose weight.

CELLULITE

There is no such thing as cellulite. It is simply a posh, pseudoscientific word for *fat*. If you have fat thighs then the best way to deal with them is to put yourself on a good diet, eat less and take more exercise. Forget about special anti-cellulite remedies.

CHAPTER TWENTY ONE

THE DIRTY DOZEN: DIETING MYTHS

When magic isn't enough

The slimming 'industry' is the biggest and most profitable part of the health care industry and many companies and individuals have made fortunes out of the twin facts that losing weight is harder than putting it on and that most would-be slimmers are on the constant look out for an easy, quick and painless way to lose weight. Everyone, it sometimes seems, wants to *lose* weight; but no one wants to have to work at it.

Here are some of the most popular diets and dieting tricks you are likely to come across — needless to say I don't recommend any of these.

MYTH 1. YOU CAN LOSE WEIGHT BY TAKING SLIMMING
PILLS OBTAINED WITHOUT A DOCTOR'S PRESCRIPTION

Millions of people buy them but I doubt if any of these would-be slimmers obtain any appreciable long term weight loss through taking them. Magic slimming pills — often sold by post — are frequently expensive but, in my view, never worth buying. Most of these pills fall into three general categories:

a) Many of the most popular pills simply contain a laxative. By increasing the rate at which the bowels work these pills can, inevitably, produce a modest short term weight loss. But after a while — or if you stop taking these laxative pills — the chances are that your weight will go back up again. The major disadvantage with these pills is that if you take them for more than a few days you are quite likely to suffer from constipation when you stop taking them.

b) A second group of pills fill up your stomach so that you don't feel like eating — or don't eat as much when you do sit down for a meal. The major disadvantage with these pills is that as soon as you stop taking them you will probably put back on all the weight you have lost (if you've lost any at all).

c) Thirdly, there are those pills which contain a diuretic. A diuretic is a substance which encourages fluid loss. In my view these pills can be dangerous because they could damage your kidneys. And, of course, once you stop the pills you will put back on any weight that you have lost.

MYTH 2. THERE ARE FOODS AVAILABLE WHICH WILL BURN UP FAT AND HELP YOU LOSE WEIGHT WITHOUT DIETING

Over the years I have come across literally dozens of 'wonder diets'. Many of them have been based on one or two particular foods which have been credited with remarkable, almost 'magical', qualities. The only way to eat a healthy diet is to eat a balanced diet.

MYTH 3. YOU CAN LOSE WEIGHT SAFELY AND EFFECTIVELY BY TAKING SUMMING PILLS PRESCRIBED BY A DOCTOR

The only truly effective slimming pills — and there is no doubt that they really do work — are the ones which are available only on prescription. There is, as you might imagine, a snag. The snag is that the most effective slimming pills in the world are probably a group of drugs known as the amphetamines — and these are extremely addictive. Many thousands of slimmers have taken these drugs,

259

become hooked on them and found that it is extremely difficult to get off them.

MYTH 4. REGULARLY ATTENDING AM EXERCISE CLASS WILL HELP YOU LOSE WEIGHT, FIRM UP YOUR BODY AND GET THE SHAPE YOU WANT

It is, of course, quite true that exercise will *help* you lose weight. But exercise alone won't enable you to lose vast amounts of weight. To get rid of one pound of fat you need to use up approximately 3,500 calories. You'll be able to see how hard it is to get rid of 3,500 calories through exercise when I tell you that even if you exercise very hard — running, for example — you will only burn up around 500 calories an hour.

During recent years I have heard claims that by doing the right types of exercise you can lose enormous amounts of weight. Exercise can help you to tone up muscles (and having toned up muscles will undoubtedly make you look slimmer) but I don't think it will make a dramatic difference to your total weight or suddenly ensure that you have a pert bottom or breasts as big and as firm as beach balls.

By all means use an exercise programme as part of a get fit programme (though do make sure that you talk to your doctor first, make sure that any exercise programme you start has been prepared by an expert and always stop if you notice any pain or discomfort).

Exactly how many calories can you burn up exercising?

The number of calories you burn up during exercise depends on several factors — including the amount of effort you put into your exercise programme and your weight — but this list will give you a rough idea of the number of calories you can expect to burn up in a 30 minute exercise session.

Aerobics: 250

Bodybuilding: 150

Boxing: 250

Cycling: 225

Dancing: 150

Gardening: 125

Golf: 125

Housework: 150

Jogging: 200

Rowing: 250

Running: 250

Sex: 150

Skiing: 225

Squash: 250

Swimming: 150

Tennis: 200

Walking: 150

MYTH 5. YOU CAN GET RID OF UNWANTED WEIGHT SAFELY AND QUICKLY AND PERMANENTLY SIMPLY BY VISITING A SURGEON AND HAVING A WEIGHT REDUCING OPERATION
There are many special operations available these days for would be slimmers who want to lose weight more or less overnight. Here are two of the best known:

Liposuction
Fat is sucked out of your body (usually from the thighs) with a tube and a piece of equipment which bears a passing resemblance to a sophisticated vacuum cleaner. The fat then collects in a jar and can be thrown away. You leave the clinic slimmer and lighter. I am

extremely sceptical about the long-term effectiveness of liposuction. I think there are better ways to lose unwanted fat.

Jaw wiring

The idea behind this particular operation is simply that if your mouth is closed you won't be able to eat very easily — and if you can't eat then you'll lose weight. The surgeon performing the operation uses steel wires to bind your two jaws together. The operation may produce a temporary weight loss but many of those who have tried it have simply put all their weight back on again when they have had their jaws unwired.

Some people have even managed to have their jaws wired and *not* lose weight. One woman I know of discovered that by using her blender she could liquidise all her favourite foods and drink them through a straw poked in between the wires holding her jaws together.

MYTH 6. YOU CAN LOSE UNWANTED WEIGHT BY GOING ON A LOW FLUID DIET

The theory behind this diet is that many people put on weight because they drink too much fluid. I doubt if that is true. In my experience most people who are overweight are fat because they eat too much food. Fluid doesn't usually pay too large a part in their weight problem. I am extremely sceptical about this type of diet. Indeed, it worries me. I am sure that anyone who goes on a low fluid diet would lose weight. But I worry that by going on a low fluid diet they might put a strain on their kidneys. Besides, I can't see a low fluid diet offering anything more than a very short-term dieting success.

MYTH 7. A NO FAT DIET IS THE BEST WAY TO LOSE WEIGHT

As the name suggests a 'no fat' diet simply involves cutting out as much fat as you possibly can — avoiding fatty meat, dairy products and other foods which are rich in fat. At first glance this diet sounds very sensible. After all, fat is well known to be a killer — it is partly responsible for the high incidence of heart disease in the Western world.

However, I don't think that cutting all the fat out of your diet is really the safe, effective way to lose weight permanently. Your body needs some fat. Without fat your hair will lose its lustre and your skin will soon become dry; more important you will become deficient in fat soluble vitamins A and D. You could even develop a serious mental disorder if you ate a diet which didn't contain enough fat.

MYTH 8. A HIGH FAT DIET IS THE BEST WAY TO LOSE WEIGHT

I have to confess that I don't have the faintest idea why this diet ever became popular. But it has, and diet experts regularly suggest that the best way to lose weight is to eat large amounts of butter, cheese, fatty meat, full cream milk and other fatty foods.

I regard this as a potentially dangerous diet. I have explained elsewhere the hazards of a high fat diet. If you followed a high fat diet you would probably develop diarrhoea. This would probably lead to a loss of fluids, vitamins and minerals and the long-term consequences could be exceedingly dangerous.

MYTH 9. A LOW CARBOHYDRATE DIET IS THE BEST WAY TO LOSE WEIGHT

Too much carbohydrate will make you fat. But too little carbohydrate will lead to dizziness, tiredness, irritability and faintness. I don't like diets which involve an unbalanced food intake. And a low carbohydrate diet is, by definition, unbalanced.

MYTH 10. A HIGH CARBOHYDRATE DIET IS THE MOST EFFECTIVE WAY TO LOSE WEIGHT

Some carbohydrates are essential but a high carbohydrate diet makes absolutely no sense at all to me. I cannot see the point of it. Your body needs a balanced diet to survive in good condition. Even if a high carbohydrate diet helped you to lose weight temporarily you would eventually have to go back to a properly balanced diet — and then you would probably put back all the weight you had lost. The only sensible way to lose weight permanently is to learn proper, sensible eating habits.

MYTH 11. THE LOW PROTEIN DIET

This diet bursts into prominence every few years. But I don't like it at all. In my view the real danger is that in order to achieve a real weight loss you would have to reduce your protein intake considerably. You would, indeed, have to lower it so far that your body started to break down its own protein stores. This, in turn, would mean that muscles would start to disappear. How do you know that your heart muscle won't be the first to suffer? In my view a low protein diet could be potentially fatal.

MYTH 12. THE HIGH PROTEIN DIET

In my view this is yet another potentially hazardous diet. I think the gravest danger with this diet is that it could put the kidneys under too much pressure. Anyone with a kidney disorder or a kidney infection might become seriously ill if they followed this diet. I think that in order to reduce the danger of kidney damage you would have to drink a lot of fluid — every day. And I rather suspect that the large quantities of fluid you would have to drink would probably mean that you might gain weight instead of losing it.

CHAPTER TWENTY TWO

TEN DIETING EXCUSES — AND WHY YOU SHOULD FORGET THEM

1. I DON'T HAVE THE TIME TO DIET

'I keep meaning to go on a diet,' is a common cry. 'I could be slim if I had the time. But my life's so busy. It's all right for her — she isn't as busy as I am.'

If dieting really did involve weighing out food portions, working out calorie values and spending two hours a day in the gym then these excuses might be valid.

But real dieting — dieting that will make you slim for ever — need not take any time. However busy and important you may be you should still be able to find the time to eat sensibly and to lose your unwanted weight quickly and permanently.

2. I'M LARGE FRAMED

I can't tell you how many times I've heard this excuse — usually coming from hugely overweight men and women who have rolls of fat bursting out through their clothes.

Bones weigh very little and add, at most, just another few pounds to your weight.

If you can strip naked, look in the mirror and tell yourself honestly that your weight problem is caused entirely by the size of your bones then I may — just may — believe you.

3. EVERYONE IN MY FAMILY IS FAT — IT RUNS IN THE FAMILY

It is quite true that being overweight does seem to run in families. But if you are fat and blame your ancestors you should know that there are two reasons for the fact that you are overweight.

First, you may, it is true, have inherited a certain genetic tendency to be overweight. But this tendency is not terribly important. Overweight is not a dominant gene. You do not always have to be fat just because your parents and grandparents are fat.

Second, and much more important, you probably learned bad eating habits from your parents when you were small. If your mother and father ate too much — and were overweight — then you probably grew up being used to the idea of eating too much. And you were probably overweight as a child. That, I'm afraid, is almost certainly the main reason why you are over-weight today.

If you are prepared to learn new eating habits — and to throw aside the bad eating habits which led to the fact that you are currently overweight — then you should be able to get thin and stay thin.

You don't have to be fat just because your parents were fat.

You can't change your height — that is something which is governed entirely by your genes — but you can change your weight.

4. MY PARTNER PREFERS ME WITH A BIT OF FLESH ON MY BONES

This excuse is most commonly favoured by women — though I've heard men use it.

It is perfectly true that most men do prefer their partners to have some curves. Survey after survey has shown that men are not sexually attracted to particularly thin women — and may, indeed, be rather frightened of them. You only have to look at the pictures in a 'girlie' magazine or to examine the paintings of nude women in an art gallery (the old time equivalent of a 'girlie' magazine) to realise the truth of this statement. If men really liked very skinny women then all the top nude models would be skinny.

But it's not generally true that men prefer fat women either.

Some do, of course. Some men like their partners to have rolls of fat, to have huge, baggy thighs and to have pendulous breasts which need restraining with brassieres designed by engineers.

And some women like to be made love to by mountainous men who have vast stomachs and fat-laden limbs.

But these are exceptions.

Most men and most women prefer their partners to be curvy rather than fat.

So, if you use this excuse take all your clothes off and stand in front of a full-length mirror. That is what your partner sees. Now, be honest: would you describe yourself as curvy or fat?

5. I LOVE EATING TOO MUCH TO CUT DOWN — IT'S MY ONLY PLEASURE

If eating food is your *only* pleasure then you need to sit down and carefully re-evaluate your life. There is nothing at all wrong with enjoying your food — but if it is your *only* pleasure then there is something sadly wrong. You need to find new aims, new ambitions, new objectives, new hopes, new aspirations.

6. AT MY AGE EVERYONE IS OVERWEIGHT

Most people do tend to put on a little excess weight as they get older. There are two good reasons for this.

First, we all tend to do less exercise as we age. We become slightly stiffer. We aren't as fit as we were. Our joints tend to seize up a little as arthritis and other disorders begin to take over. We move more slowly — and usually have the time to be a little slower.

The result is that we burn up fewer calories. And so, if we eat the same amount of food as we did when we were young the inevitable result is that we tend to put on weight.

Second, because we tend to have more available time as we grow older we tend to spend more time eating. People in their twenties and thirties are often rushing about looking after children or building up careers. They don't have much time for long lunches or leisurely evening meals.

But although these may be explanations for why people are overweight they do not provide an adequate defence.

Being aware of these hazards you should take care to watch your weight as you get older. You should be careful not to eat too much. And you should try to ensure that you take plenty of exercise.

If you allow yourself to become overweight then your whole body — joints, heart, lungs etc. — will suffer.

7. DIETING IS IMPOSSIBLE FOR ME BECAUSE I HAVE TO EAT OUT A GREAT DEAL

Many businessmen and women claim that they are only over weight because they have to spend a lot of time eating in restaurants or attending dinners.

This is no excuse.

No one forces a diner to choose the most calorie rich foods in a restaurant. Or to eat everything put before them at a dinner.

People who eat out a lot of the time can control their weight just as easily as anyone else — if they have the necessary willpower.

8. I CAN'T AFFORD TO GO ON A DIET

This excuse really is nonsense.

You don't have to buy special foods in order to diet successfully. You don't have to buy pills or attend expensive classes.

All you have to do is to eat sensibly — and to eat less.

Anyone who can afford to eat can afford to diet.

9. SLIMMING IS SEXIST — I REFUSE TO GET INVOLVED

Some women claim that dieting is an activity which is designed by men to control women. It may well be true that parts of the dieting industry are controlled by men. It may be true that many women model themselves on photographic models who are selected because they are young, attractive and fairly slender. And it may be true that the people who spend most time dieting are women.

But it is nonsense to use any of this as an excuse for not dieting.

There are two huge industries vying for our attention.

On the one hand there are the food companies which are keen to persuade us to eat more — and to eat all the wrong foods. These industries want to make us all fat — because if we are fat it will be because we have eaten too much, and contributed to their profits.

On the other hand there are the diet promoters who are keen to sell their pills and their dieting techniques. These people want us to slim (but they don't want us to stay slim because if we stay slim then we will be of no future value to them).

You should learn to ignore the exhortations, claims and counter claims of both these pressure groups.

Eating sensibly, and maintaining your weight at a healthy level, should be something you do for yourself.

Fat women who refuse to diet because they claim that dieting is a sexist activity are merely grabbing at yet another excuse for their inability to control their own greed.

10. IT'S MY HORMONES

This is the failsafe argument frequently put forward by the fat person who has tried all other excuses and found that they don't work.

It is perfectly true that some people are overweight because of hormonal problems. If you genuinely think that your weight problem could be caused by a hormonal disorder then you should see your doctor straight away. But for every individual whose overweight is caused by hormone problems I could find many thousands whose weight problems are caused simply by eating too much.

CHAPTER TWENTY THREE

DR VERNON COLEMAN'S SLIM FOR LIFE PROGRAMME

Warning: You should not begin any diet without first checking with your doctor. Successful dieting can affect your body in many ways and may alter your need for prescription drugs.

Nibbling: The Painless Way to Lose Weight Permanently

Eating three square meals a day is old fashioned and bad for you. The healthy way to eat is to eat *mini-meals*—and to eat little and often. You probably think of it as nibbling. Marketing experts call it 'grazing' because it is the way that wild animals eat. Whatever you call it eating numerous small meals is much better for you than eating just three big meals. Follow this regime and you will lose weight quickly, efficiently, painlessly and permanently — without taking tablets, performing exercises, spending money on special foods or feeling hungry.

Just look at the evidence:

* A group of doctors working in Canada have shown that nibbling is good for your health — and an excellent way to slim.

* Researchers at Tokyo Medical School have concluded that 'three meals a day are quite artificial'. They have pointed out that in contrast to big meals — which lead to fat storage *mini-meals*are burned up as soon as they are eaten.

* Researchers in America have shown that slimmers can lose two to three pounds a week while grazing, even though they may be eating 300 calories a day more than slimmers on other diets.

* Tests in Wales have shown that one group of people who 'grazed' gained no weight while another group who ate the same food as three set meals gained up to ten pounds each in just three weeks.

* Research in Chicago showed that when young children are encouraged to 'graze' and eat *mini-meals*rather than eat big set meals they grow up slim and healthy.

* Other studies have shown that if you nibble — instead of gorging yourself on three big meals a day — you will have lower cholesterol levels and be less likely to suffer from heart disease.

All the available evidence shows clearly that if you eat *mini-meals*whenever you are hungry your body will burn up the calories you consume. By spreading your energy intake throughout the day you won't ever feel hungry or faint. And you will be far less likely to put on weight than someone who eats three square meals a day.

Meals are bad for you.
Most of us eat at fixed meal-times. We eat at breakfast time, in the middle of the day and again in the evening. But as far as your body *is* concerned this is a bizarre, unnatural and thoroughly irrational way to eat. Your body doesn't just need food three times a day. It needs energy supplies all day long. By choosing to eat fixed meals you create problems for yourself.

HERE ARE THREE REASONS WHY YOU SHOULD NEVER EAT ANOTHER MEAL AGAIN:

1. When you eat at fixed mealtimes you eat whether you are hungry or not. Instead of obeying your body's inbuilt appetite control centre you eat because the clock shows that it is time to eat. Your body's internal appetite control can make sure that you never get fat — if only you let it. But eating meals at fixed meal times means that your natural appetite control centre doesn't get a chance to work properly.

2. When you eat at fixed mealtimes you tend to eat what is available, what you have prepared or what you have been given — whether you need it or not. It is easy to eat the wrong foods — and to eat too much.

3. Because you and your body know that it will be some hours before you eat another big meal there is a tendency to overeat. Your body then stores the excess food as fat so that you can live off the fatty stores while you are not eating. But because you probably nibble a little between meals your body will never need to burn up that stored fat -– besides your next fixed mealtime probably comes just before your body starts burning up those stored fat deposits.

Meal times are not natural. They were invented because they just happen to fit in with the way most of us work and live. If you get most of your calories three times a day at fixed meal times then you are almost certain to end up overweight. Calories that aren't burnt up straight away will end up stuck on your hips. And however much you try to diet the chances are that you will fail.

The best way to slim successfully is to eat small amounts of food whenever you feel hungry.

Make meals a thing of the past. 'Grazing' is healthy. And it will help you stay slim. And while you're changing your eating habits

make a real effort to eat less. Most of us eat far too much —
dangerously overloading our bodies.

Golden Rule

If you are going to try my *mini-meal* diet there is one golden rule
that you *must* remember:

Only ever eat when you are hungry

Every time you are about to eat ask yourself if you are genuinely
hungry.

If you are — eat!

But as soon as your hunger has gone - stop eating.

The *mini-meal* diet depends heavily upon you learning to
recognise when you are hungry - and being prepared to obey your
body.

Silver Rule

The *mini-meal* diet will work best if you leave between 60 to 90
minute gaps between *mini-meal*s.

What Can You Eat?

Don't be worried or puzzled about what you can eat - and how you
can eat a balanced diet without eating meals. There is no need at all
to worry. The type of food you need to eat isn't going to change at
all - just the way you eat it!

20 Sample *mini-meal*s

1. Mixed vegetable soup (90 calories)

2. Baked beans on wholemeal toast (140 calories)

3. Raw carrot with dip (70 calories)

4. Small herb omelette (200 calories)

5. Tomato salad (30 calories)

6. Low fat yoghurt (70 calories)

7. Boiled egg with slice of bread (200 calories)

8. Raw apple (60 calories)

9. Salad sandwich on wholemeal bread (180 calories)

10. Slice melon (15 calories)

11. Bowl of porridge (300 calories)

12. Corn on the cob (100 calories)

13. Vegetable pasty (230 calories)

14. Half a grapefruit (15 calories)

15. Bowl of cornflakes with soya milk (150 calories)

16. Fresh fruit salad (50 calories)

17. Spaghetti with tomato sauce (250 calories)

18. Baked potato with cottage cheese and pineapple (170 calories)

19. Grilled vegetable burger in bun (400 calories)

20. Two toasted muffins with honey (400 calories)

BONUS NUMBER ONE

The *mini-meal*diet may help to lower your blood cholesterol level. A recent American study showed that men who ate every hour (instead of three times a day) had lower blood cholesterol levels. In Canada researchers found that people who ate 17 (yes, 17!) snacks a day had less fat in their blood than people who ate identical food in three large, main meals.

Big meals stimulate the body to produce insulin to cope with the high blood sugar levels that follow. And the insulin stimulates the liver to produce cholesterol.

By lowering your cholesterol levels the *mini-meal*diet may help to protect you against heart disease.

BONUS NUMBER TWO

The *mini-meal*diet won't just help you get slim. Eating *mini-meals*will also help you to live longer.

When you start eating *mini-meals* you will soon find that you are fussier about what you eat — and you will eat only what your body needs.

By eating just what your body needs you will look younger, feel more energetic, feel sexier, avoid infections and diseases such as arthritis and live longer.

In Okinawa in Japan people eat just 40% less than other Japanese people — they also have lower rates of cancer, heart disease, diabetes and mental illness. And more people from Okinawa live to be 100 years old than from anywhere else in Japan.

Reducing your food intake will probably increase your life expectancy and reduce your susceptibility to illness.

Warning

If you are going to start the *mini-meal* diet then you must stop eating meals. You can't eat *mini-meal* and ordinary meals as well!

You don't have to be unsociable and leave your family and friends to eat alone. If they want a meal sit down with them but just eat a *mini-meal*.

The *mini-meal* diet will help take advantage of your body's central eating control mechanism.

Your body has an impressive appetite control centre which can make sure that you never get overweight or underweight. It can even make sure that you eat the right mix of foods — so that your body obtains all the protein it needs and the right mix of vitamins and minerals.

The existence of the appetite control centre in your brain was first identified in research work done by Dr Clara M Davis of Chicago in the 1920s. Dr Davis's initial aim was to find out whether newly weaned children could choose their own food and eat enough to stay alive, select a good balance of different types of food without being told what to eat and pick foods designed to keep them healthy.

The infants in Dr Davis's experiment chose excellent and well varied diets. Their growth rates, development and appearance were just as good as those of babies who had been given foods selected by nutritionists. The babies chose the right food — and just as important — ate them in the right quantities. And they stayed healthy.

Later Dr Davis reported that in an additional research project she had studied 15 infants for between 6 months and 4 and a half years and had come to the conclusion that they all were able to select a good variety of satisfying foods, ensuring that they ate neither too much nor too little. Their eating habits were, of course, unplanned and may have looked rather chaotic to the trained eye but none of the infants ever developed stomach ache or became constipated. None of the children who were allowed to choose their own diets became chubby or fat.

Subsequently further research, this time done with soldiers, showed that when adults were allowed access to unlimited supplies of food they ate just what their bodies needed. Even more startling was the fact that the soldiers varied their diet according to their environment, quite naturally selecting a mixture of protein, fat and carbohydrate that was ideal for their circumstances and needs.

The conclusion has to be that the presence of the appetite control centre means that if you listen to your body when it tells you what — and how much — you need to eat, then you will stay slim and well fed for life.'

Despite the existence of this astonishing appetite control centre most of us do get fat, of course. We eat the wrong types of food. And we eat the wrong quantities. There are several reasons for this.

Some people eat because they are depressed or anxious or miserable. They eat because they are bored. And they don't stop eating when they are no longer hungry. They become overweight — or ill — because they have overridden their appetite control centres.

There is evidence that babies who are bottle fed are morelikely to put on excess weight than babies who are breast fed. And, of course, fat babies often grow into fat children who then grow into fat adults.

The appetite control centre is directly controlled by the amount of sugar circulating in your blood and is designed to ensure that you eat what your body needs, when your body needs it and in the quantities required. Things go wrong because you ignore your appetite control centre and instead of eating according to your needs eat according to behavioural patterns imposed on you by the society in which you live.

Our eating habits are usually established when we are very small. We are taught to eat at meal times (whether or not we are hungry). We are told off if we don't clear up all the food on our plates (whether or not we need it). We learn bad habits and we learn to ignore our appetite control centre.

If you were bottle fed when you were a baby then the chances are that you started picking up bad habits before you could sit down at the table. One reason why bottle fed babies tend to get fatter than breast fed babies is that while it is impossible to see how much milk has been taken out of the breast (and, therefore, how much is left) it is all too easy to see exactly how much is left in the bottle. Anxious mothers tend to encourage their babies to empty the bottle even when their babies are no longer hungry. (In fact there is a device in the female breast to make sure that breast-fed babies do not get overweight before their appetite control centre starts to function properly. The contents of breast milk change slightly when the mother's body decides that her baby has had enough to drink. This change in the constituents triggers the end of the baby's feeding response. Breasts are far more sophisticated than most of us realise.)

These distorted behavioural patterns all help to ensure that your appetite control centre is ignored and overruled. Your eating habits are controlled not by your body's genuine need for food but by a totally artificial conception of its requirements. By the time we reach adulthood most of us have learned to eatfor all sorts of bizarre reasons. We have learned to eat when we are sad or lonely. We have learned to eat when we are happy or want to celebrate. We have learned to eat simply because it is an official meal time and everyone else around us is eating. We eat what the advertising copywriters want us to eat and we eat it when the boss says we should eat it.

However, you can break all these bad habits. And by following the *mini-meal*diet you can allow your appetite control centre to re-establish itself. By abandoning habits which overrule your appetite control centre, by learning to eat when you need to eat and by listening to your body (so that you eat when you are hungry and stop when you are no longer hungry) you will find it possible to lose weight and maintain a steady weight without following an artificial dieting programme.

CHAPTER TWENTY FOUR

FORTY EIGHT QUICK TIPS FOR LOSING WEIGHT

1. Try to set yourself easy slimming targets. If you try to get rid of all your unwanted weight in a month you will probably fail. Decide what your ideal weight should be and then aim at losing two pounds a week.

2. Remember that regular exercise will help to tone up your muscles and burn up a few extra calories. You don t have to do anything you don't enjoy. Two of the best — and most stress-free — exercises are swimming and walking.

3. Try to resist the temptation to weigh yourself every day. Weigh yourself once a week. Your weight will naturally fluctuate and if you weigh yourself too often you will be confused (and possibly even disappointed) by the results.

4. Don't let other people decide what you eat (or when you eat it). If you're full — stand up for yourself and say so!

5. Remember Coleman's First Golden Rule of Slimming: Only ever eat when you are hungry. Coleman's Second Golden Rule of Slimming is: Stop when you are full. Every time you are about to put food into your mouth ask yourself whether or not you really need it.

6. Whenever you feel hungry and you find yourself reaching for food wait five minutes. Then — if you still feel hungry — you can eat.

7. Try to get into the habit of using sweeteners instead of sugar.

8. Make a real effort to eat most of your meals sitting at the table rather than slumped in front of the television. You need to concentrate on what you are doing if you are going to use the power of your mind to help you slim successfully.

9. Never be afraid to throw food away if you don't want it. Don't eat up scraps just so that they 'won't be wasted'. Sort through all your food cupboards and your fridge every week and throw out (or give away) food that you aren't going to use.

10. Learn to let your body help you diet by deciding when — and how much — you need to eat.

11. When you sit down to a meal wait for a moment or two and relax. Then — and only then — start to eat. And eat slowly. If you concentrate you will be far more likely to hear your body 'talking' to you and telling you when you are 'full'.

12. Acquire a new habit. Try stopping between courses for a short rest. If you've had enough to eat get up and leave the table. If you stay sitting at the table after you've finished eating there is a risk that you will nibble at whatever is left.

13. Learn not to eat too much in the evening. If you eat when you are about to go to bed your body will store the unwanted calories as fat. Do most of your eating early in the day — so that your body can burn up the calories.

14. Whenever you have to have a big meal try to have a snack half an hour beforehand. The snack will spoil your appetite and ensure that you feel full long before you do your diet too much damage.

15. Make sure that you never reward yourself with food. If you want to celebrate do so with a bunch of flowers, a new CD or a book or magazine.

16. Put a little time in trying to work out how you acquired your bad eating habits. What bad eating habits did you learn as a child? Awareness of your bad eating habits will make them easier to conquer.

17. Many people who find slimming alone difficult benefit by joining a slimming club. There are hundreds of slimming clubs around. Look in the local telephone book or ask your doctor. Many people get support and encouragement from slimming with others.

18. Be prepared for the compliments when you start losing weight. Some people (particularly women) get frightened when they realise that they have become sexually attractive — they don't know how to cope.

19. Ignore 'magical' or 'wonder' diets that promise you instant slenderness. And don't waste your money on slimming pills or supplements.

20. Don't worry if you find that you need less sleep. Slimmers often need less sleep. If you have given up meat you will probably also

have more energy. A diet that contains a lot of fat often leads to a constant feeling of tiredness and exhaustion.

21. Tackle each day as it comes. Try not to think too far ahead.

22. Once you start to lose weight you will find that some people who you thought of as friends will start to scoff. They will tell you that you'll soon put back all the weight you've lost. They will do this because they are jealous. Ignore them.

23. Be positive about your new eating programme. Don't say: I'm trying to lose weight'. But say: 'I've changed my eating habits and I'm losing weight.'

24. Never forget that no one else is to blame for your weight. You have the ability to control how much you weigh.

25. Make your right hand into a fist. That is the size of your stomach. The amount of food you need to eat in order to fill your stomach would only fill a container the size of your fist.

26. See if you can find a friend who wants to change her or his eating habits — and maybe lose weight too. Ring one another up every day and offer encouragement and advice and support.

27. If you want to take up exercise do something you really enjoy and look forward to. If you don't enjoy it then you won't do it properly (if at all). Walking, cycling, dancing and swimming are four of the best forms of exercise. Remember that if you are receiving medical treatment or are in any way uncertain about your

health you shouldn't do any exercise unless your doctor has given approval.

28. Make an effort to learn how to relax — and to deal with stress. Many people eat when they are under pressure — it's an easy and commonplace way of dealing with problems. If you can deal with stress effectively there will be less temptation to eat too much.

29. Always weigh yourself at the same time of day (i.e. morning or evening) and wearing (or not wearing) the same clothes.

30. If you have difficulty in losing weight but are taking prescribed or over the counter drugs talk to your doctor or pharmacist. Many drugs cause weight gain — or make it difficult for you to lose weight. You should not, of course, stop taking prescription drugs without first talking to your doctor.

31. As soon as you start to lose weight throw out the clothes that no longer fit you. Keeping them is merely a sign that you don't expect your dieting to be permanent. This book is going to help you make sure that this diet is the last diet you ever need try. Buy yourself new clothes and slim into them.

32. If you need a break but don't really feel hungry do something else — write a letter, do a crossword, make a phone call, go for a short walk or read a magazine. But don't eat just because everyone else is eating.

33. Remember that alcohol is packed with calories. And remember that low-calorie soft drinks are available when ordering drinks in a bar.

34. Collect recipes for snacks. You'll be surprised at how many quick, tasty, nutritious *mini-meals* you can make.

35. Always read the labels on food when you are shopping. You will soon learn to differentiate between the good and the bad.

36. Make sure that you don't spend too much time looking at attractive food. You can get fat simply by staring at food because when you see, smell or think of food your body starts to prepare its digestive processes. Saliva is released and your stomach juices get ready to digest the food it expects. Your pancreas will be stimulated to produce insulin and the insulin will start to convert the glucose in your bloodstream into fat because it anticipates more food coming in. As your blood sugar level falls so you'll feel hungry. And you'll eat. Even though you weren't hungry just a few moments earlier.

37. Don't worry too much about trying to make sure that you eat all the necessary vitamins and minerals that your body needs. Just eat a balanced diet. Your body will do the rest.

38. Don't bother weighing food or counting calories. It's mind numbingly boring and unnecessary.

39. Keep one or two glucose sweets (the sort sold for athletes) in your pocket. On rare occasions only if you are feeling hungry and

don t have a snack handy have a glucose sweet to boost your blood sugar level and take away the hunger pangs.

40. Learn to enjoy your food. Get into the habit of tasting every mouthful. If you enjoy your food you'll eat more slowly and your appetite control centre will have a better chance to operate effectively.

41. When putting out food choose the smallest plate that you can practically use. If you use a big plate there is always a danger that you will fill it — and then empty it! If you have a small plate you can always refill it if necessary.

42. Turn off the telephone while you are eating. If you are interrupted your appetite control centre will probably get confused.

43. Always chew your food properly. If you chew properly then you will be less likely to suffer from digestive upsets and because you will be eating slowly you will give your appetite control centre a chance to work properly.

44. Always put down your knife and fork between courses and stop eating for a while (though if you are on the *mini-meals* diet this won't really apply). This will make sure that your body has a chance to tell you that it is full.

45. Eat as many raw vegetables as you can. They take a lot of chewing but are better for you. Because they take a lot of chewing they will slow you down — and give your appetite control centre a better chance to work.

46. If you buy fizzy drinks always buy the diet 'low calorie' versions.

47. If you must eat biscuits buy the small packets — with just two or three biscuits in them. They are expensive but you're less likely to end up eating half a large packet in five minutes.

48. Don't worry if your good intentions slip occasionally. Don't give up your new eating programme just because you misbehave for one day. Just start again the next day.

CHAPTER TWENTY FIVE

CHILDREN WHO ARE OVERWEIGHT

A lifetime of obesity and dieting often begins in childhood. Children who are fat often stay fat — and find it extremely difficult to lose excess weight later in life.

How to cope if your child is fat

At least one in four children is overweight. Obesity is now one of the biggest health problems facing children.

Children who are overweight are likely to:

* grow up to be fat adults
* develop heart disease
* develop high blood pressure
* develop chest problems
* develop bone and joint problems
* develop diabetes
* find exercise difficult
* suffer from more colds and coughs
* suffer from anxiety and depression
* be victims of bullying at school
* suffer from loneliness

The vast majority of overweight children get fat because they eat too much — or eat the wrong foods. It is rare for a child to be fat because he or she suffers from a hormone or glandular problem.

You can help your child get slim and stay slim.

But you must take care.

If you push too hard you could make your child anorexic. Remember that pound for pound growing children need twice as many calories as adults. A child who weighs just five stones will probably need as many calories as an adult who weighs ten stones.

Many of those extra calories are needed to help the child grow.

Twelve ways to help children lose excess weight — and stay slim

1. Never push them into eating up all the food on their plate if they say they are full. If you are worried that they aren't eating enough talk to your doctor. If you push children into eating more than they want you could make them fat for life by teaching them bad eating habits.

2. Try to teach them the facts about foods. You will be surprised at how interested most children are in what they eat. Explain why fresh vegetables and fruit are good (they're full of vitamins and fibre and low in fats) and why chocolate and cake are bad (they are low in fibre and vitamins and full of sugar and fat).

3. Remember that many children overeat because they are looking for love. Give children plenty of love and they won't need to nibble on bars of chocolate to cure their unhappiness.

4. Be consistent. And be fair. Don't advise your children to cut down on the chocolates and then let them see you pigging out on a whole bar of chocolate. If you are overweight thenyou too should try to control your weight. Your children will find weight control difficult to understand if they see their parents eating anything and everything — and ignoring their own weight problem.

5. Encourage children to eat slowly. Fat children often eat far too quickly. Teach children to chew properly. And remember that good table manners will help keep weight down.

6. Remember that breast fed babies are probably less likely to become fat than bottle fed babies.

7. Don't use food as a punishment or a reward. If you do then your children will associate food with emotional as well as physical needs.

8. Make sure that children have a good breakfast but eat as little as possible in the evening when calorie requirements are at their lowest.

9. Encourage children to eat when they are hungry whenever possible. Do not allow children to read or watch television when they are eating. Children who eat while doing something else will not be aware of their appetite control centre. They will just keep cramming food into their mouths automatically, regardless of whether or not they are still hungry.

10. Try to keep children out of the habit of eating lots of sweets. Sweets ruin the teeth and are usually rich in calories. Teach children to understand which foods are fattening.

11. Encourage children to take regular exercise. Too many parents insist on carrying their children everywhere by motor car.

12. Weigh children regularly. If they seem to be gaining weight too quickly then try to correct this. It will be easier to make a modest

correction now than to try to deal with a massive weight problem in a year or two's time.

We hope you found this book useful. If so we would be grateful if you would post a favourable review on Amazon.

Vernon Coleman is a qualified doctor and the author of over 100 books (including *Bodypower* and *Spiritpower*) which have sold over two million copies in the UK and been translated into 25 languages. There is a list of his books on his author page on Amazon. Many books by Vernon Coleman are available as kindle books on Amazon. For more information please visit http://www.vernoncoleman.com/